Love and Loss

The Storied Nature of Nursing Home Care

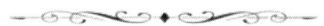

Carolyn Bailey Lewis, Ph.D.

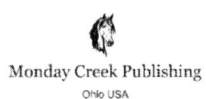

Monday Creek Publishing
Ohio USA

Monday Creek Publishing | P.O. Box 399 | Buchtel, Ohio USA
mondaycreekpublishing.com

1. Family Relationships 2. Eldercare 3. Later Years 4. Life Stages

Dedication

To my loving, stellar, and attentive daughter Caryn Michelle Bailey who sacrificed her career in Washington, D.C. and relocated to Ohio to become the greatest support and advocate a person could have. Without her love and care, all would have been lost.

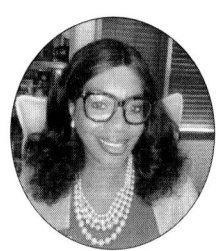

"I have one mother and didn't think twice about moving to Athens to take care of you. Nothing else mattered. My love for you is infinite so, above anything else other than God, my choice will always be you. When you were at death's door, I felt hopeless and devastated. I prayed and prayed and prayed and asked God to give me the desires of my heart because you, Mom, had given up." I said, "God, I feel like I'm constantly asking for something because I know You always supply my need according to Your riches in glory. But right now, I need You to do this as she is the matriarch of my family and my best friend. I need her here." All the while as I, her mother, felt my body drifting to another place, I was praying, "She needs me, Lord." God heard our prayers and remained faithful. I'm still here.

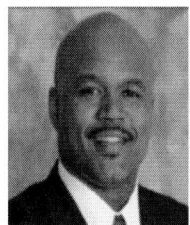

I am grateful for the enduring love, wisdom, and concern of my son Carey Isiah Bailey who demonstrates purpose through his life and career, my two granddaughters Evann and Leah, their mother Angela, and my late husband Bob Lewis who epitomized love through my sickness and health.

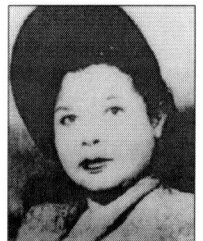

Great Aunt "Mama" Thelma Stone. Because of you, I am.

Contents

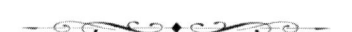

Acknowledgements

Thank you to Caryn my daughter and Samorra Dower for their work in transcribing several of the interviews, Rose Dikis and Dr. Dianne Bouvier for initial proofing, friends Brad Stalnaker for the cover and Dr. Patrice Harris for her review. I could not have made this journey without the prayers and support of numerous relatives, friends, and colleagues.

I am thankful for the work of the wonderful medical providers and staff over the years who attended to my care. I planned to express appreciation to each individually, but the list kept growing and I feared I would omit someone. I will simply say "Thank You" to the doctors, nurses, aides, therapists, and staff who have been crucial to my healing journey, and to the fine health care providers at J.W. Ruby Memorial and Monongalia General Hospitals in Morgantown, West Virginia; Camden-Clark and St. Joseph's in Parkersburg, West Virginia; OhioHealth O'Bleness Hospital in Athens, Ohio, Charleston Area Medical Center in West Virginia; and OhioHealth Riverside Methodist Hospital in Columbus, Ohio. The health care providers saved my life several times with quick and decisive action. Special thanks to The Laurels in Athens, Ohio; Dr. Jacqueline Nicholas, Riverside; Jim Reeves, CNP, Fairfield Medical Center in Lancaster, Ohio; and Dr. Christopher Edmands, Parkersburg, West Virginia.

In addition to The Laurels, I express gratitude to HealthSouth Rehabilitation in both Morgantown and Parkersburg, West Virginia, Washington University's Barnes-Jewish Rehabilitation Center in St. Louis, Missouri, Ohio Valley Health Care in Parkersburg, West Virginia, and Kimes Nursing and Rehabilitation Center in Athens. Each experience was unique, sometimes disheartening, yet instructive.

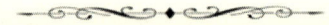

Introduction
Insider

I write as an insider and a trained journalist who has stayed at six nursing homes and physical rehabilitation centers, and seven hospitals, a period of 26 years. I had developed mobility issues from a benign spinal cord tumor in 1995 and have experienced ups and downs in working to regain strength and to walk again. Three times I've had to learn to walk and it's been an incredible journey, to state the obvious. I have had to learn to do everything all over again – several times – from writing my name to typing, dressing, showering, eating, turning over, balancing, standing, walking and, once, talking.

Even though I lost control of bodily functions and felt helpless at times, I never lost my faith or my strong mind. My son Carey told me once, "Mom, use your mind. You've got a good one. Your body will catch up." I certainly had to remember that and keep it in the forefront when, following months of recovery in 1995 from an 11-hour spinal cord operation in Morgantown, West Virginia, I returned to work to lead the television staff. It was especially important in 1997 when I relocated to Athens, Ohio, where I was back on my feet when I applied for the position of general manager of the station walking and started the job three months later in a wheelchair. "Use your mind."

From observations and conversations, I learned that everyone in nursing care has a story, including me. I have several, especially backstories, and so do others. I was a "curious" insider. My only nursing home knowledge before my illness was as a visitor and, now, here I am. My journey includes seven hospitals with various stays – five in West Virginia and two in Ohio. In addition, I received physical rehabilitation at a facility in Missouri where Christopher Reeve (also known as "Superman") was treated for paralysis following a horse-riding accident. There were five more times at nursing home and rehabilitation centers – three in West Virginia and two in Ohio. Medical providers, therapists, doctor office visits, emergency transports, surgeries, out-patient care, and home health? Too numerous to count.

Although regulated by state laws, the quality and standards of nursing and rehabilitation facilities vary. My first rehabilitation facility was superb. It even had a therapy pool. I progressed exponentially with mobility and walking. The second and the third facilities were excellent, too. Both helped me get back on my feet following return bouts of paralysis. The accommodations of the fourth facility were dismal and the physical therapy was only so-so, but the food was phenomenal. The fifth was a mistake where I received pressure sores due to negligence and though my daughter and I gathered documents to file a grievance, we learned we did not file within the appropriate time frame. I should have selected the sixth facility before the fourth and fifth. It was the cleanest and most spacious with a lovely room, excellent therapy services, and manicured grounds. Even with my setbacks, the sixth facility became my healing home and one that felt more like family. It wasn't until a neurologist in Columbus properly diagnosed my issue as Neuromyelitis Optica (NMO) and regulated the medication that I stopped having so many health reversals.

I have experienced harrowing events over the course of the past 26 years – the 11-hour laminectomy (the removal of a portion of the spinal canal roof) and removal of the spinal cord tumor that precipitated it, paralysis, extensive rehabilitation, falls at home, a transient ischemic attack (TIA/mini stroke), mobility issues, low potassium, the NMO, plasma exchanges by the Red Cross, two life flights, three blood pressure falls (40 over 10, 50 over 20, and 48 over 20) when my normal pressure was 116 over 67, intensive care several times, blood transfusions, medicine transfusions, high white blood cell counts, feeding tubes, sepsis (life-threatening organ dysfunction triggered by infection), gall bladder removal, kidney stones, bleeding on the brain, urinary tract infections (UTIs), three pressure sores (one almost infected my tailbone), and a femur break when I bent over trying to put my shoe on.

I would have been dead, and should have been, if not for the Lord on my side, excellent health care providers, and supportive family and friends. I wanted to be home, in my bed, and would have been except for the setbacks. I gratefully say – but God. His grace and mercy, and prayers of the prayer warriors have kept me not only alive, but alive and flourishing. Purpose.

You readers who know me and rarely saw me miss a beat, because I kept pressing through every situation, are probably saying, "Who knew?" A person with whom I serve on several committees said she never knew anyone who could get as much accomplished as I do while dealing with such adversities, from a nursing home room.

My daughter would not let me give up even though she was experiencing illness herself and from which she has been healed. One evening in 2017, I was almost gone. I was not eating or drinking water, regurgitated any medicines given to me, and was having a negative reaction to Rituxan infusions (used to treat certain autoimmune diseases) for the NMO. The infusions, every six months, took six to eight hours. Normally 180 pounds, my weight dropped to 128 pounds. Caryn walked into my room that evening and said, "Mom, have you given up?" I was so weak that I just nodded my head. She said, "You have," and left.

The next thing I knew, my daughter returned with five or six women led by a stalwart Athens community prayer warrior and elder. I actually thought this visual was heaven. I knew several of the women and they were powerful in prayer. Had the rapture come? As she neared my bed, the elder repeated, "You shall not die, but live, and declare the works of the Lord! You shall not die, but live, and declare the works of the Lord!" (Psalm 118:17). Not only did I live, she said, "By Sunday, I decree you shall be eating." I had lost 52 pounds and was nearly skin and bones. That was a Thursday. By the following Sunday, three days later, I began to eat and eventually the feeding tube came out. She spoke the Word.

How one gets better depends on the degree of love and support – family, church, friends, and community, plus personal motivation. It was definitely all of those on that "you shall live" night. Those women probably didn't realize the lasting impact they made. They dropped whatever they were doing to see about me. I'm eternally grateful.

Early one morning in 2018, while wrestling with God over why I wasn't progressing as quickly as I thought I should and why I was in my sixth facility rather than in my home, I clearly heard, "You're the journalist, there's purpose. Write the story. "What?" I said. "Write the story." Yes, I am an insider who happens to have mobility issues and who also happens to be a journalist. I am an insider who, while healing and undergoing therapy, observed, participated, and listened. Then, I was inspired and compelled. I interviewed. I researched. I wrote. I am declaring the works of the Lord. Purpose.

A Scary Proposition

It's scary. *You* think about it. "As I grow older or become disabled," you contemplate, "who will care for me and what will be the level of that care?" "What will happen to my home and to my possessions?" "What will be the cost?" "How will I pay?" Much is written and discussed about nursing home care. Over media, lawyers assert they will "find the truth" about what happened to a loved one – a fall, a bruise, or even death. I've observed that the majority of falls are caused by the residents themselves who think they can do more than they can. One of my dear acquaintances was transitioning to death but thought she was strong enough to get up and go to the restroom by herself. As soon as she stood, she fell and broke her hip.

The statistics are staggering and what we read and hear about most skilled nursing homes are the negatives. Not all stories, though, are heartbreaking. Some are lifesaving. Love. Others express abject sorrow. Loss. I find it difficult to understand family members who abandon their loved ones, especially those who live close to a facility and don't visit or contact their people. It's close to criminal. Others don't bother to call. Perhaps it is fear of their own mortality or even guilt. I've watched the loneliness, lonesomeness, and the rapid demise of people who have no contact with family. It's a rapid down-hill decline. You might not have a family member or friend in the hospital or in a facility, but you would brighten someone's day if you would seek out those without support and fill in the gap for them. You might not be able to do everything, but you can volunteer and do something. Each one, reach one.

This book will illuminate some personal stories and provide examples of the underpinnings of nursing home structures. I never experienced or saw physical abuse, although I know it occurs. Close to verbal abuse? Yes. There are a variety of ways one can be abused – staff not answering a light, leaving a resident in distress; staff refusing to assist a colleague with a resident; malnutrition, or staff withholding service from a resident they don't like. I pointed out to an aide that a resident lashing out is usually not about the aide but about the person's frustrations, although I firmly believe what poet Maya Angelou said, "Even when I have pains, I don't have to be one." Displacement from one's familiar surroundings into a foreign environment is disorienting and causes confusion. Therefore, residents retaliate verbally and sometimes physically to express unhappiness with the living situation. However, staff must be kind and compassionate or find another profession.

Indeed, abuse is prevalent in myriad nursing homes in countless ways. In addition to narratives of love and loss, I offer "insider's" advice for policy and practice, and the significance of having an advocate and advocacy. Caring must be intentional in the wider framework of nursing and rehabilitation. I have frequently said to a caregiver, "Treat residents as if each was your favorite grandmother or grandfather."

The hub and happy place for any nursing home is the activities program. In later chapters I delve into the dynamics of Bingo, volunteers, and therapy dogs, with focus on the importance of listening physicians, caring nurses, attentive aides, focused therapists, activities, cleanliness, and dietary quality. All are woven throughout the tapestry of narratives. Through my research, I found nursing home stories seen through the lens of counselors, psychologists, and social scientists, yet none from a "curious insider."

What follows are true, both my own lived experiences and first- and second-hand accounts of love and loss gathered through interviews with residents and/or family members, and health care providers. One story is told by a daughter, speaking as if she were her mother. She recounts, through her mother's lived experience, what it was first like to watch her husband spiral down the dark staircase of dementia and then to experience the same herself. Someone once said when you lose a person with dementia you lose them twice, once when they are diagnosed and then when they die. This is called "Ambiguous Loss." A rapidly shrinking brain is how doctors describe it. As the patient's brain slowly dies, they change physically and eventually forget who their loved ones are. Patients can eventually become bedridden, unable to move, and unable to eat or drink.

What's to come is a compilation of my experiences in several facilities.

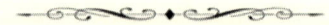

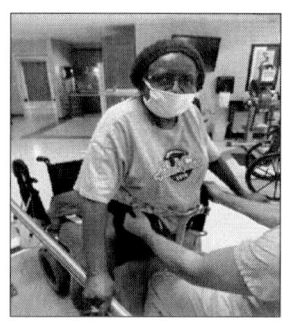

The author in parallel bars

Chapter 1 – What Am I Doing Here?

I never imagined my life would take the turns it did. I spent those 26 years off and on as a patient in hospitals, doctor's offices, skilled nursing homes, and rehabilitation facilities. About 30 years ago, a young woman who sang in a Gospel choir with me had to move into a nursing home. I think back and realize I thought at the time, "Surely this is the end for her." I was wrong. I hadn't been in such facilities myself because of age, mental lapses, or displacement. I still owned my home and possessions. Yet, I can't count the times I asked myself, "What am I doing here?" while batting balloons in therapy with folks who were "pleasantly confused," placing pegs in holes, and participating in activities that seemed mindless to a younger patient in facilities where there were 80- and 90-

year-olds. Though it wasn't the end, it was different and difficult. Sitting in physical, recreational, or occupational therapy, and even with a counselor in psychology sessions (where I ended up counseling him about his issues) with octogenarians (as a 50 something), was disheartening.

At times, I was living two lives. Parallel lives. During most days in my later years of inpatient rehabilitation, I was "out and about," going to athletic events, movies, shopping, church, events on campus and in the community, going to meetings, visiting friends, going home two or three times a month for a few hours, taking and initiating conference calls and Zooms, attending committee meetings, helping others and doing paperwork, teaching an online class – you name it – all while doing therapy five days a week. In essence, my office was my skilled nursing home room. Who knew? My pastor had his secretary make a sign for my door that reads, "'Room and Office of Dr. Carolyn Lewis." I even teach the online college class right from my room with my laptop. At night, it was back to bed at rehab. A resident could go around the world but had to be back to check in before midnight for insurance reasons, personal care and pharmacy needs, and to keep the room. I always joked when I was out that I had to be in before midnight or I would turn into a pumpkin.

So, you ask, why have I been in and out of rehabilitation for so long? The primary reason is regaining and maintaining mobility in order to function more independently. Because my spinal cord took such a hit from the tumor, there have been lesions and issues emanating from the surgery. The secondary reasons were the pressure sores – easy to get and difficult to heal. I had three large ones when I arrived at the sixth facility. Two are healed and large one is healing but stubborn. I am almost there and finally understand that it takes protein to aid in the healing process. One of my nurses kept saying, "protein, protein, protein" until I finally believed her. The sore on my coccyx grew to the size of a large fist. At the time of this writing, it's the size of a dime. Shearing, or slight tearing or abrasions, has often been a concern, also, because the skin gets thinner and more subject to damage the less mobile one is.

My entire situation could have been depressing and would have been for many people. Especially trying were times when I needed assistance doing almost everything. This sixth go around is taking an exorbitant amount of time for me to heal and to regain strength. A therapist asked me, "How do you keep from being bitter after all you have been through?" I told her it was my deep, unshakeable, abiding faith in God and in the work of Jesus on the cross. I Corinthians 15:58 says, "Be steadfast, unmovable, always abounding in the work of the Lord forasmuch as you know your labor is not in vain in the Lord." And it isn't about me. It's about Him.

Every situation was another opportunity to witness as to how my roots run deep in the Word because of experiencing the ever present love of God and knowing my life, with all of its bumps and bruises, has purpose. To me, it wasn't what was occurring that mattered. It was how I dealt with each event. My singular job was to keep my eyes on the prize knowing that someday, one day, my living will not have been in vain.

Years ago I heard a young man give a testimony in church, saying, "I'm going to the grocery store to witness and to share the love of God and, while I'm there, I'll get my groceries." Purpose. Few people knew the "rest of my story" insofar as where I was spending my days and evenings most of the time – in rehab. God in my life made the difference along with family and friends. Through it all, I never lost my faith, my joy, my temperance, or my peace. I can't say the tears did not flow sometimes or that I didn't get lonely for my home, being with my daughter, and having my independence. It was tough. A plaque in my bedroom reads, "Remember to Pray." When I would get through my mini pity party and pray, my strength would be renewed.

Navigating the decision to enter a nursing home is agonizing. Often, there is no other choice. My being in such homes has never been because I didn't have my own home or needed a place where I would live out the remainder of my life. In essence, no one was "putting me away." Again, my status has been physical and occupational rehabilitation due to mobility issues. Residents who are unable to care for themselves at home and must turn to a nursing home often feel abandoned and ashamed. The other option is home health care which can be expensive, depending on insurance, and uncertain if you don't have an aide who is trustworthy and reliable. One resident told me, "My family put me here, I didn't want to come." And another, "My family has taken all of my things and put me here." Of course, we know of horror stories about patient care (or non-care) and many of those accounts are undeniable. There are some extremely sad stories, yet stories of love exist as well as those of loss – stories we need to hear.

As a now 73 year-old woman with a vibrant, ever curious, and learning mind, I occasionally feel lost, though, in the midst of loss. I ask myself again, as the Bingo numbers are being called, and seemingly mindless residents wander the halls, murmuring – lonely and lonesome – "What am I doing here – still?"

I repeat the same therapy processes, more intense each week, over and over as the days and months speed on. I look around, and ask, "What am I doing – here?" In all of my illness journey, interestingly enough, I never asked God, "Why?" I was more concerned about the "what." I work hard at therapy and stay involved with as many of the activities as I can. I stopped playing Bingo for a while because I saw it as a waste of time, not realizing how much the game increases socialization, memory, and hand/eye coordination. My Bingo story comes later. I thought I should be doing other, mind-challenging things. To be in the midst of so many residents who could not communicate, were confused, or were unable to remember their names and those of family members, or even where they were, was quite disturbing.

I could see the love and the care of most nurses and aides who hugged residents, carefully arranging their clothing or their hair. Forlorn, empty looks were evident, yet some residents exuded hope and anticipation of getting better through therapy and returning home. Me.

While constrained to therapy and healing, I found myself helping others, praying with them, singing and ministering in the weekly church services, and being an advocate. I realized meaning when, because of my witness for Christ – not with words only, but with my actions – nurses and aides would ask me to pray for them or their families. I thought about my own situation and asked the Lord, "Who am I to pray for them when it's obvious I have so much to deal with myself?" The answer was clear. "Who are you not to pray when you have been anointed to do so?"

I sum it up in one word: Purpose.

And we know that all things work together for good: to them that love God, to them who are called according to His <u>purpose</u>. – Romans 8:28

Chapter 2 – The State of Care

A pastor and author said to me, as I was giving him the premise of my book, "America is one of a few countries that does not embrace the elderly." And I add, often has distain for those with disabilities. In several of my Communication and Media courses, I have had a number of international students. During some of our conversations, I learned their primary purpose was to get a good education in order that they might go back home and take care of their parents to pay them back for their sacrifices. They emphasized their parents would never be in a nursing home.

According to the Centers for Disease Control and Prevention (cdc.gov), nursing homes are a type of long-term care facility for people who do not need to stay in a hospital but, for medical reasons, cannot live on their own. Most nursing home residents are elderly, but younger adults with mental or physical disabilities may also stay at such facilities. In the United States, the majority of nursing homes are certified by both Medicare and Medicaid, though a decreasing number are certified by only one or the other. There are approximately 15,600 nursing homes and 1.7 million licensed beds in the United States, of which 69.3% are for-profit. Nursing homes vary significantly in size and about 2,022 nursing homes in the U.S. have fewer than 50 beds, while around 6,900 have between 100 and 199 beds. Nursing home facilities employ over 1.8 million people, with over half being aides and attendees.

The State of California has the highest number of nursing homes of any U.S. state with 1,219 facilities, followed by Texas and Ohio with 1,212 and 951 respectively. Alaska has the fewest but has the highest annual cost for a private room in a nursing home. A private room in an Alaska nursing home costs $297,840 per year on average, while a private room in Connecticut, the second most expensive state, costs $160,600 per year. Some nursing homes have special care units for patients with Alzheimer's disease or serious dementia, diseases common among the elderly. Such patients can require special or increased care. Almost 10% of all nursing home beds in Colorado are Alzheimer's special care unit beds, highlighting the demand for such care.

The elderly account for the vast majority of nursing home residents in the U.S. The largest share of residents are aged between 85 and 94 years, accounting for one third of all residents. Women are at higher rates than men, with around 11.2% of all women over 85 years living in nursing homes, compared to 6.1% of men in the same age group. Common medical issues among nursing home residents include bladder and bowel incontinence, depression, weight loss, and pressure sores. Additionally, around 36.6 % of all nursing home residents have severe cognitive impairment.

It is notable that women live longer than men and are more apt to be caretakers, to care for husbands or partners at home rather than place them in a nursing facility, or even to enlist a home health aide. A friend told me she was exhausted taking care of her spouse and felt she owed it to him to let him remain at home, even though her own health was deteriorating. There is a fine line when making health care decisions. The solution? Be informed, explore every angle, and make sure the caretaker's health does not suffer in the admirable process of caring for another. By all means, know you can't do it alone. Get help, take respite or time away, and allow space for yourself to rest and restore.

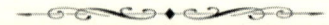

Chapter 3 – Nursing Home Laws

With an increasingly aging population, according to the U.S. Census Bureau, the U.S. has seen a consistent rise in the number of Americans living in senior living residences, including nursing homes. Approximately half of Americans who reach the age of 65 will need long-term living services. With an increase in seniors living in nursing homes comes an increased awareness of the issues that face those who live there.

For the most part, elder abuse laws are handled at the state level. Most of these laws were developed in the 1980s and are found in a variety of state legal codes. Since the Older Americans Act was put in place in 1965 in order to increase the standard of living for Americans over 65, the legal system has responded with laws related to the abuse, neglect, and financial exploitation of the country's elderly citizens. The elder abuse issue faces nearly one in 10 American seniors. As more

21

Americans report abuse in nursing home care, the legal system must respond with laws and regulations that help protect the rights of elder citizens.

State Regulations on Nursing Homes

Residential care facilities are typically licensed and regulated at the state level, with every state having at least one legal category for residential care. While many states' laws and regulations cover the same general areas, their contents tend to vary considerably from state to state. For example, training and staffing requirements are handled differently from one state to the next. Ten out of 50 states have no direct care worker training requirements. Of the states that do, the number of training hours ranges from one hour to up to 80 hours of staff training.

The Centers for Medicare and Medicaid Services introduced requirements for service providers, including all long-term care residences that are paid through Medicare. As a result, many states will be required to amend their laws in order to satisfy the minimum requirements of these services. This includes regulations on choice of roommates, access to food, personal privacy, planning requirements, and more issues regarding personal autonomy.

State regulatory provisions cover a wide range of nursing home topics, including: Residency agreements, policies on admission and retention, disclosure requirements, service planning, requirements of third-party providers, medication delivery provisions, food and dietary regulations, requirements of staffing and staff training, background checks, provisions for dementia care, inspection requirements, and state regulations.

Some elements of nursing home laws are more consistent from state to state. Nearly all states have regulations on residency agreements and specific requirements for what must be contained in these agreements. Thirty-nine states also require Disclosure Statements, whereby a facility must provide detailed and complete information to prospective residents about their potential place of living, but only 16 out of those 39 states provide a template that the care facilities must follow.

It's important to know your state's laws for what qualifies for residence in a particular living facility and what conditions must be met in order to retain residence. For example, state laws regulate how promptly payments must be made, the level of health you must maintain to qualify for certain facilities, and more. It's crucial to know your rights and the rights of your family members so you can sufficiently prepare for every stage of life. States don't vary too much in the scope of services they allow nursing homes to provide, but they do differ in the details of services they must provide. These provisions cover things as frequency of laundry and housekeeping, how transportation must be handled, and how often services must be available. Only six states do not require facilities to provide three meals per day.

One major point of variation is how nursing and medical services must be administered. Some states do not allow nursing homes to furnish full-time nurses, whereas other states require that full-time nurses be on-hand 24/7. Some states allow nurses to delegate nursing tasks to unskilled or unlicensed staff members, whereas 15 states require a licensed healthcare professional to administer all medications.

Another significant difference among states is the staffing ratios or numbers required and the degree to which staff must be trained. If residents in nursing homes are receiving insufficient care or are victims of neglect resulting from understaffing or poorly trained staff, they can consult their state's laws to know if they have the right to demand a higher level of care.

States also differ on the degree to which background checks are performed which can result in a lack of safety in states that don't have sufficient provisions. The risk of elder abuse increases when background checks are not required.

Side Bar: The Nursing Home Reform Act is the main policy outlining federal nursing home laws. The Act was first implemented by the U.S. Congress in 1987 and created guidelines for long-term care nursing homes receiving federal Medicaid and Medicare funding. Federal nursing home laws under the Nursing Home Reform Act cover aspects of nursing home care from resident rights to staffing and operational requirements. Under federal nursing home laws, the health and wellbeing of residents may not decline unless medically unavoidable.

Federal nursing home laws state that residents are entitled to receive:

- *Medically related social services*
- *Proper health care, such as primary and dental care*
- *Accurate dispensing, receipt, and administration of medicines and drugs*
- *Dietary services that meet daily nutritional needs of each patient*
- *Special services for mentally ill or mentally impaired residents*
- *Personal, material, and financial privacy when requested*
- *Treatment that does not violate the resident's dignity or respect*

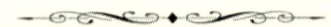

Chapter 4 – Skill Nursing - Lifeline

Twenty-first Century nursing is the line holding a patient's health care journey together. Across the entire patient experience, and wherever someone is in need of care, nurses work tirelessly to identify and protect the concerns of the individual.

While nurses are skilled, not all provide the same level of care. I have encountered nurses who appear to not want to be bothered. At one facility, I waited over an hour for a nurse to attend to my wound care while I was wet from a shower. An aide told me the nurse was doing paperwork. When the nurse finally arrived, I asked her which was more important, paperwork or patient work? I was so disturbed that I really didn't want her to help me further, but I had no choice. She was the only one on duty and, thus, the exacerbation of my wound issues.

I've encountered a few harsh nurses, too. I get a slow boil for two reasons: When I hear a resident spoken to with less than kind words and when a nurse comes to my room to tell an aide help is needed in another room. I want to say, "If you took the time to come in my room to tell the aide help was needed elsewhere, why didn't you take care of the concern?" I have overheard abrasive words to residents and reported the nurses to management because no one deserves that treatment. One of the aides mentioned to me, and I can't claim credit for the idea, that one or two nurses and aides should be hired to go undercover such as a secret shopper or an undercover person on some of the television reality programs. All nurses should be aides first to fully understand what aides encounter and endure. Often overworked, underpaid, and always under mandates (involuntary extension of one's work hours based on a vacancy in the next shift), there must be a better way for the aides' shifts to be filled.

Beyond the time-honored reputation of nurses for compassion and dedication, for the most part, lies a highly specialized nursing profession which is constantly evolving to address the needs of society. From ensuring the most accurate diagnoses to the ongoing education of the public about critical health issues, nurses are indispensable in safeguarding public health.

According to the American Nurses Association, (nursingworld.org) nursing can be described as both an art and a science; a heart and a mind. At its heart lies a fundamental respect for human dignity and an intuition for a patient's needs. This is supported by the mind, in the form of rigorous core learning. Due to the vast range of specialized and complex skills in the nursing profession, each nurse will have specific strengths, passions, and expertise.

However, nursing has a unifying ethos: In assessing a patient, nurses do not just consider test results. Through the critical thinking exemplified in the nursing process, nurses use their judgment to integrate objective data with subjective experience of a patient's biological, physical, and behavioral needs. This ensures that every patient, from city hospital to community health center, state prison to summer camp, receives the best possible care regardless of who they are, or where they may be.

In a field as varied as nursing, responsibilities can range from making acute treatment decisions to providing inoculations in schools. The key unifying characteristic in every role is the skill and drive that it takes to be a nurse. Through long-term monitoring of patients' behavior and knowledge-based expertise, nurses are best placed to take an all-encompassing view of a patient's wellbeing.

All nurses complete a rigorous program of extensive education and study, and work directly with patients, families, and communities using the core values of the nursing process.

In the United States today, nursing roles can be divided into three categories by the specific responsibilities they undertake. When diagnostic results come in, the nurse reads them first and, if necessary, immediately notifies the appropriate doctor. Gone are the days when nurses acted like the doctors' handmaidens. Today, nurses are equally responsible for the overall care of the patient. Regardless of the facility, the same nursing processes are utilized – scientific methods designed to deliver the very best in patient care, through five simple steps: Assessment, diagnosis, outcomes/planning, implementation, and evaluation. Nurses are key to the health of a nation. I've had nurses (and aides) who simply would not leave me or leave the facility if I was in distress, until my daughter and the doctor had been notified, and I was stable or headed for the hospital. Several times nurses made split-second decisions that saved my life. Nursing is a calling, not a vocation.

Chapter 5 – Nursing Aides: Heart, Soul, and Backbone

Facilities tend to literally break the backbone by not caring adequately for the aides; not being compassionate about their working extremely long shifts with heavy loads; not helping them balance family, school, and work; being inflexible during family crises, such as a birth, death, or operation; being indifferent to who is scheduled, where, and when; and not understanding the need to be considerate, even after the scheduled shift has ended. Good aides are forced to quit for the lack of empathy or for being treated and spoken to as "less than."

Believe me, aides know more about residents than the doctors and nurses – our moods, concerns, complaints, hurts, and issues. They see the tears, care for the lonely, and attend to the deceased. They are seemingly the lowest rung on the care ladder, yet have a mountain of responsibilities and are the ones to whom others should listen – especially when they observe and report a marked change in a resident. Their pulse (no pun intended) is constantly on the residents because they are in and out of residents' rooms more than any other provider in a facility. They should not be dismissed because they don't have degrees. Aides do more than bedside care. They offer support, comb hair, shave beards, paint nails, hug, listen, and just help make residents feel better about themselves. And yes, they do all of the dirty work, too. Aides are the first responders to call lights. Again, nothing peeves me more than to see lights blinking and nurses running around trying to find an aide (who might be busy in another room) instead of answering the call.

I was told by an administrator that no staff – from housekeepers to administrators – should pass by a room with a light on. They might not be able to help, but at least stop to make sure the resident is not in distress until the aide comes. Wishful thinking.

Points of Advocacy
- *Increased salary and benefits for aides*
- *Every aide should be evaluated on individual performance and resident feedback,*
  not just an across the board "meets requirements."
  State Tested Nursing Assistants (STNAs) must be more than warm bodies. They must be thoroughly in-

*terviewed, checked, and trained for the specific facil-
ity. Every facility has a particular culture, and every
resident has different requirements and procedures.
No matter how long a person has been an aide, one
size does not fit all.*

Residents have to develop a trust factor for aides; distrust comes when aides lie to residents, steal, treat them roughly, speak harshly, won't listen, push back on requests, or don't own up to mistakes – nurses, too. When aides act as if they know everything when a resident is trying to explain how care should be, no bond can develop between them. Those who hire aides must have a sense of their suitability for the work, not just because they are needed to fill a spot. Training on real people, not just dummies, is a must. I've offered to be one on which new aides could train and kiddingly offered be placed on the payroll for all of the training I've provided. My question to a new aide: "You've never done peri-care, a foley, or changed a colostomy?" Aide: "No, only on a dummy." Me: "What?" My first thought after such conversations is, "We're in trouble."

Excellent aides are pushed for more work and criticized by others; slackers get by. Some aides and nurses have attitudes that limit care received: "I'll answer your lights if you are my buddy," "I'll help with your treatments because you're my pal," or "I'm not going in Dr. Lewis' room, she's too picky." Who are they to decide? Another issue I have is when aides ask others for help on their halls, but when someone else needs help on another hall, there is no one to be found or to respond. Who suffers? The residents. And residents deserve better. They (or insurances) are paying the salaries!

I make these suggestions to new aides: Be timely; care for residents as you would your loved ones; be respectful of residents and of their possessions; be gentle; be kind; be a team player; don't ignore call lights; and don't disappear. I could write another book about abuses of breaks (consistently taking longer than permitted) which, ultimately, cheats the system and the residents.

Let me tell you about two aides I'll call "Frick and Frack." Frick could not be found when it was time for my personal care. He was in his car on his phone and he was late several times to my care. Frack lied about the care he supposedly gave me. I caught him in that lie. I have been known to be particular about my care and I don't apologize for that. However, I give any aide at least three chances and then I am done. I would never fuss, curse, yell, or scream – I'd simply say, "We're done." Then I would request another aide. Frick worked for quite a while and left or was fired; Frack was relieved of his duties.

Then there was the Alpha aide telling the other aides what to do as if he were the boss. One evening, he decided that the aide on my hall should not help me to bed because it was close to dinner, even though the nurse told her to help me. Dinner was 30 minutes away; helping me would only take 10 minutes.

My advocate, my daughter, just happened to stop by. Due to the wounds, I was only to be up in my wheelchair for so long. My daughter learned what happened and told the aide, "Don't you ever make decisions about my mother's care." He didn't again. Enough said. She has appeared unexpectedly when "interesting" situations affecting me are occurring. Problems solved. She is such a supporter of my return to good health that I would be asked by nurses and aides, "When is your daughter coming?" Most times, I really didn't know because she would pop in morning or night. Some of them didn't want to see "Ms. Bailey." If you want to know the reality of a loved one in a facility, make unannounced visits, day and night. My daughter would often visit at 3 a.m.

Aides have a reputation for quitting when the going gets rough. How can one quit a job on the spot and be re-hired without question? There is no sense of loyalty or patient care when one quits before duty ends. Isn't that abandonment? When employees walk off the job or call off incessantly, let them go – for good! If they are rehired, they know they can get away with just about anything and return over and over. No accountability. However, excellent aides should be appreciated and rewarded. Passionate aides tell me they worry about "their people" when they are away and want to make sure we are cared for and well looked after. That's commitment.

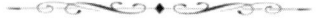

I Am <u>Not</u> a Nurse

But I show up every day for report.

I'm *not* a nurse. But I wash my residents daily and do full body inspections for anything "new" or for skin break down.

I'm *not* a nurse. But I know all my residents' diets, meals, likes and dislikes, textures, and who's a choking risk. I feed my residents who can no longer feed themselves.

I'm *not* a nurse. But I apply medicated, doctor-ordered creams and ointments, compression stockings, and safety equipment.

I'm *not* a nurse. But I do colostomy, ostomy, and catheter care.

I'm *not* a nurse. But I take full sets of vitals for them and specimen samples for labs.

I'm *not* a nurse. But I chart any changes in a resident's daily behavior and health.

I'm *not* a nurse. But I give them the answers they're looking for when the doctor asks how the resident is responding to a new medication.

I'm *not* a nurse. But I tell them how a resident's day is going while they are on the phone with a family member.

I'm *not* a nurse. But I tell them which resident is which when they're doing a medicine pass.

I'm *not* a nurse. Yet, I'm the one they come for when they need help getting blood from an aggressive resident.

I'm *not* a nurse. Yet, I am the one who gets a resident in bed, changed into a hospital gown, and ready for the paramedics to come.

I'm *not* a nurse. But I'm the one who gives them a report on residents at the end of the day.

I'm *not* a nurse. Yet, I'm the one who will sit with a resident who is scared, upset, or lonely.

I'm *not* a nurse. But I hold residents' hands, wipe away tears, and put smiles on their faces.

I'm *not* a nurse. But I do their nails and curl their hair.

I'm *not* a nurse. But I sign for hourly breath checks, sheets, and turning schedules.

I'm *not* a nurse. But I open the windows while I wash their bodies and wrap them in a shroud.

I'm *not* a nurse. But we line the hallway and say a prayer while a body is wheeled out.

I'm *not* a nurse. But I go to the wake and tell residents' families how sorry I am for their loss and how much we will miss them.

I'm *not* a nurse. But I worked 40+ hours a week during COVID-19 to care for the sick and be there for residents who are looking for their family to see them through a window.

I'm *not* a nurse. But I spend time away from my family to take care of yours.

I'm *not* a nurse. My residents have names, not just a number down the hall.

I'm *not* nurse. I see it all over Facebook.

However, I *am* a State Tested Nursing Aide.

And even though we are constantly being torn down, we still show up.

So no, if you ask, I'm *not* a nurse.

Source: Facebook, anonymous posting

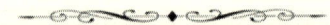

Chapter 6 – One Aide's Story

"I would tell a new aide to treat everyone with the utmost respect, let residents know the patient's rights, make sure they have a copy of the rights pamphlet, make sure checks and changes are done appropriately and, if someone has to be fed, don't set their tray in front of them and make the resident wait until you return."
– Aide C. (an aide who prefers to remain anonymous)
State Tested Nursing Assistant – STNA)

Well, to start at the beginning, I was very fearful of this line of work. I think it takes a very strong person to start in this field. You see a lot of things that are unexpected that you would not normally have to deal with in regular life. At the very beginning, I was scared. I did not understand a whole lot and I was more afraid of hurting someone. I think it is a strong point when you start in this kind of work. You are afraid of moving a person, lifting them up, or transferring them because you are afraid of breaking an arm or a finger. You are afraid of contact with people because of illnesses you do not know they have or not. It takes a long time for you to build up to a point of understanding the likes of this life and that you should not be so fearful of those things because you can control them. Now, I think I have a more balanced understanding because of how long I have worked in this field. You get accustomed to those things.

Falls come with understanding. Most times when you are new, a fall will likely happen because you are not thinking of every little thing that could possibly cause that fall. So, a newspaper on the floor is a huge fall risk, especially if it is on linoleum, because there is no friction. One foot on that newspaper, that's the end of it. Not using proper body mechanics or using gate belts properly can cause a fall. Being aware of your surroundings is critical.

You can prevent falls only so much. There is going to be a time that it happens regardless. So, if I am in a room with a person and it's happened before and they have fallen and I was there, at this point if I am close enough to them, I would lower them to the ground with my own body in a way that is not catching them per se. Because if you catch them, you are going to hurt yourself and the other person. So, you want to hold them, and kind of like hug and lower them to the ground to prevent them from any further injury. But, if it is a fall and I have walked by it and they have already fallen, I would call the nurse and let them know that a set of vitals is needed first and foremost and, from there, they would assess the situation.

Believe it or not, I never thought about being in the nursing field. My mother was a nurse, but I was always so scared of it because I saw her experiences through nursing school. She would sleep with her eyes open because of how grueling the classes were. At the time, she was working as an emergency room nurse, with a 40-hour work week, and she would have this cold-hearted attitude about everything in life. I understand where that comes from now. When I was younger, I never understood it because I was always like, "Why is my mother so cold?" Understanding the way you have to work in this field, there is a point where people do go numb if they do not know how to handle things properly. I think she just now started warming up. I never thought I would get into it. When I finally did, it was a proud moment where I wanted my mother and father to see of me. It made them proud that I jumped into this field. I was in the State of Ohio and, weirdly, you do not have to have your certification or your state test and license to be a nursing aide. For about four years, I worked without my certification. Recently, I finally got it. I love this kind of work. I really do.

I feel like, maybe it is me tooting my own horn here. I feel like no one else can do the kind of work that I can do. They can't give the kind of care that I can give. I love making people smile and happy every day. I have always been this kind of awkward type. I make jokes at myself all the time. When I work in this kind of field people get that and they enjoy it more because they are already feeling at their lowest, too. So, when I poke fun at myself, then it is more like, "Oh, I don't feel so bad for my shortcomings, too." I love that. I also love working with Alzheimer's patients over a long period of time. They know who I am and get adjusted to me. I think we need more compassion in this field.

My mother would work in nursing homes because she was once an STNA. I've gained a lot by working with people in skilled nursing. I feel, as a person, once you hit rock bottom is when you start gaining the most. After my initial shell shock of starting, I came to a point in my life where I was starting to grow numb to the routine. Everyone has to get to that point to kind of understand why you are feeling that way. At the time, I did not understand that you really do need a support system when you are living or working in these facilities. You need a positive group you can talk to and let things out in the open. I would get close to residents and see them die. I would have to hold all that in. I went by the book. I had to hold it all in and then I didn't understand why I would lash out more. I would get angry more. I would get upset more and then it all kicked in why. I was not dealing with it in a very healthy or positive way. That is not something on which we are educated. When you go through classes or do this work without getting a certification, you don't understand how to open up and say, "I lost this person, I was close to them, and I worked with them, and I loved them." Instead, you have to kind of be, "Well, they are gone."

There is a process with this. Let's say Sam died. I was there and witnessed his death. I would be the one cleaning up his body. This is a tedious process. The teeth are cleaned, body washed, and bedding cleaned. When someone dies, their body releases everything. I have to make sure all that is cleaned, their hair is combed, and they are in a nice outfit. The family will either come in shortly to view them or the funeral home will come and pick up the body. At this point, this is when the STNA will pretend the resident is only sleeping to cope with them dying. The aide knows they are dead, but they have to deal with this process like they are sleeping. That way, when the family comes in, I can say, "Well, he was really a wonderful person."

The thing they don't really tell you is that when a family member dies, there are many responses the family is going to exude. They are either one, out for the family's money which I have seen before and is really hard; or two, severely angry and screaming at the STNA for any and every reason. It is not that anything wrong has happened, but this is how they deal with their grief. And three, they cry uncontrollably and will not give space with the death. If the family came in hours before and then the resident died while they were there, it is hard to go in and clean up. There are a lot of things we have to deal with, so it is very difficult for us to be emotional about the death. That's why we have to separate our feelings in that moment. Then we have to find a quiet space to kind of let it out without family or friends seeing it, let alone our own co-workers because we do not want to bring them down, too. We have thousands of things to do every day and that is the last thing we would want.

For me, I have figured out that going to the bathroom for five minutes, crying, and then putting on a smile again is really effective in these moments. If it is really bad, on my half hour lunch, I will cry my heart out in the car and call someone who is really close to me who will just listen. We can go to funerals but, in this line of work, it is more likely you will have to work on that day, so you won't be able to go to the funeral or see them. You have to find your own way of letting go.

I miss my grandfather for sure. He struggled with cancer for 14 years. You would see him get worse then better, worse then better, and he was just kind of a fighter that way. He always had nurses and nurses' aides to come and see him. It seemed to get worse and worse every time I saw him. He would start forgetting my name. He forgot how to use the bathroom properly and was using my grandmother's purse. He would throw her shoes in the microwave. This is what happens with aggression. That was way before I became an STNA. At the time, I did not understand it and was angry. This was someone I was close to for years and he was like my own father when I was younger. My dad was not particularly close to me then. Seeing someone I loved go through this illness and seeing nurses and all come in, and how he would be so angry at them when they would come to clean him up, was so hard to understand. For one, why would someone want to clean up my grandfather?

This did not make sense to me until later. It is hard to understand why someone needed cleaned up when you are not in the field. People need to be clean. I guess when you can make logical sense of things and you have natural control of your body, it's like, "Oh, I can shower whenever I want but, when I was younger, I did not see it that way." I was thinking he can make his own decisions. To see him get so upset, your automatic response is defending your family member or loved one. It was very hard for me to understand that, but now I totally get it. Well, I have been in that situation, where lots of people say, "No I do not want it." Then I say. "Yes, you have to have it. It is important."

I have worked in this field for eight years. My mom had worked in it for so much longer. My mother would tell me horror stories but would give me the "light" version as she did not tell me what I know now. We talk about it and it is really funny how we interact lately because it is different. Well, before I was an STNA, I was a Resident Assistant and my first experience was with a home health aide company for mentally re-tarded (a term used then) and developmentally disabled (MRDD) residents. I did not know what MRDD meant at the time. There was a lot of abuse I did not understand, not on the residents, but on the aides who came in. The game completely changes at that point. You can go to tell residents that what they are doing is not cool, but if they come swinging, you cannot fight that or protect yourself. My mother told me stories about this back in her day and it made me laugh. She would take pillowcases and put her hand underneath the pillow, holding the pillow to block the blows. You cannot do that anymore, because the residents can get hurt. So now, you are the punching bag. There is not much you can do about it.

That was a shell shock to me. At that point, I was not really doing anything. I was not cleaning anyone up or helping them go to the bathroom. I can only imagine that it's far worse now. Getting them to drink water instead of soda, they would come and swing at you. I quit several jobs because of that. I was scared. I did not want to upset anyone. Even if that was the right thing for them to do, I still did not want to do it.

Then I moved on to another facility. I loved that place for their rehabilitation. I did the rehabilitation side for a year-and-a-half because I loved helping someone's knee recover or hip recover, taking them on longer walks, or letting them sit down, having a cup of coffee with them, or talking for a bit. I loved it, but I did have my first fall there. He was someone who was recovering from a hip injury and had broken his hip four times. He was doing fine walking, but I made a fatal error. I have never talked about this. I was young and dumb. We were walking to the bathroom without a gate belt. He was brushing his teeth in the bathroom and everything was good, I turned my back for a second to take off my gloves and up against the wall he went. It was that fast. I was crying because I did not know what else to do. So, I lowered him down the best way that I could. He had a dent on his arm from the light switch. All he could say is, "Before you get the nurse, put the gate belt on me so you do not get in trouble." That's what ended up happening. The nurse took his vitals and everything was fine. He did not break a hip, thank God. All he had was a shear. It took four of us to lift him. I was shocked. What's crucial, it was gate belt every time. Lesson learned.

Everything has to be a certain way now with safety. Safety comes way before comfort. I would rather someone be a little bit uncomfortable in order for them to be safe. It is just personally how I am because I would never want to experience that again.

My mom has told me things like this, too. I worked at an assisted living facility for almost three years and that was different. Coming from nursing home care, everyone has all the things they would need in their own home, and it makes it easier to find things at that point. The nursing home was trickier, depending on which hall you worked. The rehabilitation was really well organized; you could find everything with ease. They had their own shower room and people had their own bathrooms, so it was far easier to deal with things like that. But, on the other halls, it was much harder to have organization, people were stressed out. There was not enough staff and it was very stressful.

The place I worked for three years was called an "assisted living facility," but it is not. It is a nursing home. The scariest part about it though, the nursing home where I worked previously paid $12.50 an hour for an STNA, plus shift difference which could be 50 cents to $1.00 more. Assisted living paid $8.45, which is minimum wage and you are learning under somebody who does not have their own STNA. So, in that facility, they do not really want people to get their STNA because they would have to pay them more.

You see a lot of different politics with different places based on how much money the company themselves can get. It is very scary what these companies will do and there is no law against it, which is even scarier, right? When you think about it, an aide has to work with up to 40 people. One aide to 40. Brushing teeth alone is five minutes, for 40 people, that is about 200 minutes. That's about two hours of work and you only have an eight hour shift. That is just teeth brushing alone. You are not talking about bathroom, showering, or getting people to bed. A lot of places are like that. That nursing home was like that because it was understaffed.

With home health care, you really do not have to worry about that because you are the only provider. If you need two people to assist the home patient, now you have a problem. There is only one of you and not two people there, so that's a huge issue. In the assisted living facility, there were two assistants for 40 people. Technically, you would need four to five people to help with that 40 people, and there are no laws on that, right?

I think this one where I am now is a lot better – a lot. It is one of the best facilities that I have worked. I am not just saying this because I work here, but I really like it. It is much more organized, not that I can implicate a system. But we still have staff situations where we do not have enough time for a two-person assist transfer. So, what do you do at that point? Can you find another person? Are you now behind? Are you now held over? On the evening shift, that tends to happen a lot. Luckily with me, I have made friends with the people I work with, so when I need help with someone, they will help me, and then I will help them with someone. Teamwork is crucial. I know for many other people that is not the case. They will do things alone and that's really scary.

The cleanliness level is awesome. To compare and contrast, at the assisted living facility I had to clean people's rooms, do the housework, and wash dishes. I had to take people's food from the kitchen to them. I had to do their laundry on top of everything else an STNA has to do. Which, if you think about it, is a lot of contamination. Not only on my own uniform, but with my own hands and arms. There is no sure way to handle something like a major illness at that point, because there is so much cross-contamination. You are playing with bleach and other chemicals when you are doing the housecleaning. Where I am now, we do not have that problem. Everything is completely in different sections. You have housekeeping. You have a laundry department. You have STNAs. You are not forcing everything into one role. So, I really like this place. You have the tools you need here, too. You have extra Hoyer lifts. You have extra batteries. You have enough sit to stands. You have physical therapists in a gym. You don't have that in most places.

I am a seamstress. I put on events for the local community, for low income families. They usually can't do anything that costs. I am in a Steam Punk Group. We dress up in Victorian costumes that we make. I'm not to corset speed yet, but I am getting closer. We would make these costumes and be kind of goofy. At the assisted living facility, I would go to meetings dressed up this way and, before the meeting would even start, I would walk around rooms and just brighten people's day. I would really dress up for Christmas. I would wear antlers and things or Halloween and, if I could get away with it, I would wear cat ears or a cattail while I am working. I just don't see life any other way.

I will play pranks with people sometimes. I will get the tiny stir stick straws, but I will have the actual straw in my pocket. Then I will say here is your straw, then the person would say, "Well I want an actual straw." I am like, "No, that is the one you are stuck with." Then, I will pull out the actual straw and give it to them.

The reason why I wanted to do this, I talked to my mother some time ago because I wanted to do activism for STNAs. We do not get paid enough for healthcare or mental support. Healthcare benefits through companies, if you are lucky enough to get it, doesn't help with the care costs of seeing a psychologist if needed. It doesn't compensate you if there is a loss. These are things that should be in play. Most companies do not have enough people on the floor to help them. That's dangerous. Paying minimum wage is insanity and just crazy. They could fire people for no reason when I was at the assistant living facility. This is just not right. I know nurses have a nursing organization they can go to if things get really bad. They have their own union. If anything should be out of the ordinary, they can go to them and they have coverage. My mom and I looked online to see if there is a group for STNAs and there is not one. I have been looking at starting a group like that and protesting and doing what I can to change this field. My mom also said this is so similar to how she did it back in the day. "It only takes one person to start and that's me."

I would love to be an STNA a lot longer. The only problem is people don't think this is a career. Higher-ups and government people do not see this as a career. If you think about this logically, how many Alzheimer's patients like seeing the same person? You would want the same person day in and day out to be there, so that way they get on the same routine and know what's going on and get used to that person. Why wouldn't we want to interact with that? Why wouldn't we want to have that? This is why I want to do more fighting for the STNAs. In this society, honestly, there are many people out there who deserve more respect than what they get. I think it is a huge workforce that is the basis for nursing alone. You still need them in the emergency room. The ER is now hiring STNAs. Why? Because they know they need them. They know they need that type of care. It is the basics, the backbone, of nursing care. Why are we not being treated and paid better? Why aren't people being treated that way? You want the best quality care you can possibly give and they can possibly get.

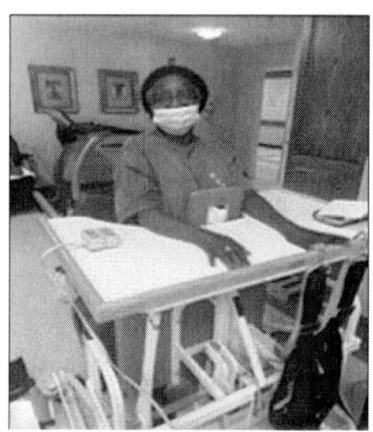

The author at a standing frame

Chapter 7 – Physical Therapy: Footing and Foundation

If STNAs are the backbone of skilled nursing home care, then therapists are the footing, the foundation. For grass to grow, the soil has to be tilled, watered, fertilized, and seeded. Though you watch, you won't see the actual growth, but the blades eventually spring up. Such is therapy. It's not easy and you have to be determined to do what is asked of you by the therapists. Believe me. They know. The same processes are repeated, with variations, as you progress. Like grass growing, you don't see or feel the immediate results, except for tightness or pain in areas on the body that have been dormant. One day there are marked results if you are persistent and remain motivated, where you can see improvements just as you would visualize a beautifully manicured lawn. Somehow, out of our seemingly flawed body – out of the soil – comes beauty and strength.

I've observed residents who don't want therapy and just want to be left alone. They balk at taking medications and just want to go home. They don't realize that the more therapy they get, the better the body responds. Then, there are others who enjoy the warmth, the 24-hour assistance, prepared food, and comfort and prefer the facility over home because of what's awaiting there. So, the blemished logic is, "If I don't do therapy to get better, the longer I can stay at the facility." According to Joint Ventures' History of Physical Therapy, physical therapy (PT) addresses the illnesses or injuries that limit a person's ability to participate and function in activities of daily life. The first to practice physical therapy are thought to be the physicians Hippocrates and Galenus. As early as 490 B.C. they advocated manual techniques and hydrotherapy for treatments. Machines were later developed to treat ailments for routine and systematic exercise of the joints. Henrik Lang, the Father of Swedish Gymnastics, founded the Royal Central Institute of Gymnastics in 1813 for massage, manipulation, and exercise. The Swedish word given to physical therapists is sjukgymnast – sick gymnast. So true. I call my physical therapist "maestro" because of the new ways conjured up to stretch my abilities. I look at her sometimes and think, "What else will she imagine?" It's all good, though. Every session, I am given a new "score" that helps my frame, and increases my flexibility, strength, and control. Physical therapists, who were once known as reconstruction aides, evolved through a series of changes to become the present ever-growing confident and accomplished professionals in the health care system. They play a very important role in providing rehabilitation and habilitation services as well as prevention and risk reduction training.

With the end of the 19th Century came the beginning of modern physical therapy. When polio became epidemic in the U.S. in 1916, physical therapy enabled muscle testing and re-education on the muscle which would increase and return functionality. Physical therapy was solidified during World War I when women were assembled to rehabilitate injured soldiers.

Walter Reed Army Hospital in Washington, D.C. opened the first physical therapy school during World War I. Research was instrumental to the PT movement. The American Women's Physical Therapy Association, formed about this time, and eventually became the American Physical Therapy Association. It currently represents nearly 80,000 members in the U.S., ranking as one of the country's top and desirable professions

I overheard a resident complain about "this place" while waiting on her physical therapy session. I rolled next to her and quietly asked if she had been to any other rehab facility. She said, "No." I told her I had been to several others and, overall, where she was now is one of the best. She was a chronic complainer, but after I suggested that she be a bit more grateful for where she was, her complaints didn't altogether stop, but there weren't as many – at least about physical therapy.

I have had to learn to walk several times because of setbacks. Physical therapy is hard, but it's worth every minute. It pushes you to the limits. Then, all of a sudden, improvement! When I was completely paralyzed from the neck down by the spinal cord tumor in 1995, I had to undertake the tedious processes of placing pegs in holes for developing muscles; remembering how to turn over; struggling to sit, balance and stand; learning to walk heel to toe, and the list goes on – all to regain strength, endurance, and confidence. It took faith, persistence, and perseverance. Kudos to the patience and love of therapists who always give those two words of encouragement, "Good job!," even when you are at the brink of tears.

Chapter 8 – Occupational Therapy: Readiness for Regular Life

Occupational therapy (OT) is a relatively new profession in which therapists work to increase skills related to work or independent living. Occupational therapy's past is difficult to determine, writes Michael Moninger in a myotspot.com blog about the history of occupational therapy. In the 18th Century, patients suffering from mental illnesses were considered a threat to society and the majority of them were simply stuck in prison and hidden from society. Human rights abuses began to surface and society looked for more humane ways to provide treatment. One development, though certainly far from perfect, involved asylums where the mentally ill could freely engage in their meaningful occupations. In these spaces, a greater degree of emphasis was placed on work and doing tasks that were helpful in life. Public Law 94-142 guaranteed children a public education and removed them from asylums which prompted the need for occupational therapy to assist with the transition to "regular" life and education.

In U.S. cities and towns, sheltered workshops that employed people with mental and developmental disabilities began to emerge. They were effective, but still separated the disabled population from others. The benefit of occupational engagement was understood more and more and participation was encouraged along with arts and crafts. The National Society for Promotion of Occupational Therapy, a professional association, emerged and is now The American Occupational Therapy Association (AOTA). The AOTA advances OT practice, education, and research through standards setting and advocacy (aota.org).

I was initially confused about the difference between physical and occupational therapies. I quickly learned the difference when the physical therapists put me to work on balance, standing, reaching, turning, walking, upper and lower body strength, and bending and reaching. Occupational therapists worked with me on developing core strength for showering, dressing, hand/eye coordination, work and home skills and, the one I like the most – cooking. Physical and occupational therapists frequently work together on various aspects of one's therapy plan. It's a team effort. In essence, PT works to strengthen the body and OT focuses on developing skills and strength to interact within the environment.

Each therapist uses unique treatment processes that are separate from other medical treatments. Instead of duplicating physical therapy's approach, OT pulled from myriad places to develop the most beneficial way to help clients' functionality. Both PT and OT involve all aspects of care giving – nursing care, social work, psychiatry, orthopedics, and more. Everyone usually knows everything about you all of the time. If you have an eye problem, a headache, or just don't feel up to par, the issue is documented and discussed by your team. The therapists, nurse, and others in your individualized care plan (ICP) develop a solution and get to the root of the matter. Therapists work with you one-on-one and can discern whether what you say you are able to do matches what they see you are able to do.

In recovery, everything has to be thought through. Many of you reading this will get up and go about your regular life without thinking about how you are going to move or function. For those working to regain functions, it takes thought and work. Occasionally, an aide or a nurse will enter my room and, when I ask, "How are you doing?" I will hear, "It's rough" or "I'm having a bad day." I say, "Hold it." I want to say, "Shut up," but I don't. I offer this, as I point to the bed and around the room: "You are not in here; you are walking, can see, hear, and talk; you have a job; you're not in therapy; and you are not six feet under." ("Shut up!")

As OT became more established, the profession and its principles spread around the world. The implementation of occupational therapy assistants (OTAs) served as a catalyst, greatly increasing the availability and ease of access for OT services.

Changes continue to be made because of recent advancements in occupational therapy. Additional treatment models are being developed as more progress is made. Although physical and occupational therapies are the most well-known, other therapies play critical roles in restoring the body, mind, and spirit: Speech, pool, psychological, restorative, recreational, music, pediatric (children), geriatric (elderly), orthopedic (muscles), cardiovascular (heart), pulmonary (lung), vestibular (vertigo or dizziness), neurological (brain and spine), and feeding or eating therapy. Each of these requires a significant amount of education and training for a practitioner to be certified and/or licensed.

Chapter 9 – Activities and Volunteers: Staying Connected

If nurses are the lifeline, STNAs are the backbone, therapy is the foundation, then the activities department and volunteers are connectors – providing residents the link with each other and to the outside world. I'll explain.

All too often, residents have no visits from family members or access to the personal touch or to the world beyond their care facility. Activities staff and volunteers bring much needed love, communication, attention, and connection to people unable to experience these things from their relatives. These staff members and volunteers enhance the lives and experiences of those who have support and undergird others who have been abandoned by family and friends. Loss.

Volunteers more often than not fall under the auspices of a facility's activities department. The activities staff, in some

form or another, usually see each resident every day –
whether passing on reading material or mail; overseeing spiritual services and entertainment; playing games; organizing
Bingo; taking residents shopping or on sightseeing trips; setting up movie hours, puzzles, painting, coloring, arts and
crafts, picnics, or cookouts; planting gardens; or building
birdhouses. A special treat was organization of a family parade
around the facility during the COVID lockdown when family
members could drive around the facility and residents could
be outside and wave from a distance. It was emotional boost
for those who had not had a glimpse of family for months, except seeing them outside the window.

Community members and students help fill in the gaps
with visits, calling Bingo, reading to residents, and overall assistance. Volunteers go through a training program and orientation. The activities department and volunteers regularly
go far beyond the call of duty to keep the residents' minds active and engaged. Puzzles, coloring pages, word find, painting,
playing cards, and trivia are among the favorites, and games
where one could win a dollar.

Individuals and groups who come in to sing, dance, or
otherwise provide entertainment are always welcomed at
most facilities. A detailed schedule is produced every month
of who is coming, what is occurring each day, and where activities will be held. A Daily Chronicle is distributed daily with
historical information and fun facts. Everyone always looks

forward to the summer cookouts when family and friends can join in the festivities. Socialization during these activities is instrumental to the well-being of residents. It keeps them feeling some sense of normalcy. Love.

One of the activities that surprised me the most was the Pen Pal Project in the summer of 2020. Residents were asked if we wanted a pen pal and I said, "Sure." They used our individual photos with a white board beside us on which our interests were written. I had them write, "Serving God, Gospel music, Jeopardy!, reading, and writing." Well, I thought our photos and interests would be sent to a local civic club or two and they would send cards occasionally. Little did I know, even though I signed the permission form, that we would be on the facility's Web site and would go viral.

Within two months, I had received nearly 60 cards, letters, and photos from Oregon to Massachusetts, Georgia to Minnesota, and everywhere in between. I answered them all. After a little over a year, about 10 pen pals and I still maintain regular, monthly contact. Most of the letters I receive are handwritten, and two to three pages long. One of my favorites is an "almost four year-old," as he wrote in his first letter, from North Ogden, Utah. He loves dinosaurs and sends me beautiful pictures he designs and colors. He is faithful in responding and I commend his mother for teaching him the valuable gifts of writing and communicating at such an early age to bring joy to another person's life.

The Nursing Home Reform Act of 1987 says all nursing homes shall provide a comprehensive activity program designed to meet the physical, mental, emotional, psycho-social well-being and personal interests of each resident. Activities shall be provided based on the needs and preferences of each resident as identified on their comprehensive assessment and care plan, as required by rules of each state.

A resident said she had been in her room for months without outside contact. This is where volunteers are valuable – to seek out those needing a good conversation and some fresh air outdoors or to read and play music to keep their minds stimulated. Some residents might just need a listening ear. Nursing homes rely on volunteers to provide a sense of place and regular interaction. You might be surprised at what you have to offer – young or old – because your very presence will make a difference. Although "nursing home" suggests nurses provide care, neither they nor the nursing aides can do it alone because there isn't enough time in the day. In fact, federal law requires any facility receiving financial support from Medicare or Medicaid to have at least five percent of the care provided to residents through volunteer workers (cdc.gov). All a volunteer needs are a caring attitude, concern, the ability to interact with others, and the desire to provide company to residents. Volunteers also enjoy assisting with other activities, even calling Bingo!

Though not all facilities are receptive to religious services, various churches and ministries of all denominations regularly visit facilities to offer their services including a service (usually on Sundays and Wednesdays) and visits throughout the week. Two people who volunteer their time each Sunday and almost daily in a facility are Pastor Barry and Mrs. Lynne Bolin. He conducts services, officiates at funerals, marries, and administers Holy Communion. Lynne teaches a weekly Bible study. They both visit rooms and pray. Residents can have affiliate membership with Romans Road which is chartered to the facility. According to Pastor Bolin, it started with Margaret H. who knew him when he was working at a mental health center. He tells the story:

Romans Road Church – A Unique Volunteer Ministry
From the perspective of Pastor Barry Bolin

"I said I would agree to start regular church service and we could call it the 'Romans Road to Heaven' Church."

Margaret heard I was providing pastoral work for many nursing homes and teaching adult seniors Sunday School in a church. I visited her on a couple of occasions when she was a resident in another facility. She was a short-term resident there for physical therapy. After her husband passed away several months later, she somewhat declined in health. Several months after a new facility in Athens opened, she went there to live. She liked it so well she submitted an appreciation for the local paper to print about the place for new skilled nursing and rehabilitation.

I do not recall exactly when, but I believe it was in January 2012 when Margaret called me to see if I would volunteer to come to present devotions to the residents. After discussions with her about this, Margaret set up a meeting for me to discuss it with the activities director. I agreed to be a volunteer and completed the paperwork. She wanted devotions to be on Sunday mornings if I would do them.

We set 11 a.m. on Sunday mornings to have devotions and I believe we started in February 2012. In addition to my Sunday School teaching, I was reading and studying the Bible daily, and I did my own research of different doctrines of many denominations. I remember well the first Sunday I had two people other than Margaret for devotions. The next Sunday that doubled to six and I then started to make visits to the facility on Mondays to talk to other people and each Sunday more would come until we had about 12 people attending regularly.

The activities director, Margaret, and I started discussions on actually forming a church service. I believe the activities director felt that she needed to have a church set up for residents. I told her I was much interested in studying the Book of Romans and did take studies at a university. I said I would agree to start regular church services and we would call it the "Romans Road to Heaven Church."

On August 28, 2012, I was ordained as a licensed independent minister. A few months later, I was given the "Laying on of Hands" and I use Romans 8:28 as my Scripture for witnessing to many people. Margaret and I discussed with the activities director, since I was an independent minister and studied doctrines of other denominations, that no other church services would be scheduled Sundays which would confuse people for many different reasons. She agreed and stated she would need a person to do devotions on at least one weekday. Over the years, I've found pastors to do this. My wife Lynne felt led then to help with devotions and now, she is holding devotions every week. It's called "Devotions with Lynne."

Well, back to Romans Road. It continued to grow until where we had 20 or more attending with eight to 10 different denominations with that few people. We not only had long-term but also short-term people attending from all walks of life – short-term meaning post-hospital or post-surgery people there for rehabilitation therapy. By this time, four people started promoting other people to come to the church on Sunday. I talked with them that maybe we should try to charter the church.

After research, I found out I did not need to do this for state regulations for a couple of reasons – mainly we were not receiving collections or asking anyone to give and no one was paid for this service. We were still able to get the church chartered by the National Association of Independent Ministers and they chartered us in the Year of Our Lord 2014. They declared, "There is a need for ministry that the herein named organization is providing in the promotion of Christian faith; therefore, it is granted the recognition of this independent ministry at the Romans Road Church Service at the named facility of Athens in care of Barry P. Bolin.

Actually, Lynne and I were fully taking care of all expenses. A couple of outside people said they wanted to help us, so I set up a Romans Road bank account. A few donations were given here and there, and Lynne and I sat down after prayer and decided to give monthly ourselves.

By this time, there were many expenses for different things, such as Communion and printing of the hymn sheets. I was also making visits to several places including Columbus hospitals on a regular basis to do pastoral work with people from the facility or other nursing homes. We supported the church with our money for these expenses along with other expenses such as paper for songs, ink for printers, sound system, and cards for various occasions. We even set up a video system which we never had to use. There were expenses for Daily Breads that they use, ink pens, calendars, snacks for food on certain holidays – the list goes on. So, a couple of donations received did help.

In February 2015, I typed a membership form for people to join. The reason? So that they could say they were members of a church in order that the date of membership would be on it and be known. I included a birthdate where we could celebrate their birthdays in the Romans Road Church service, their favorite Bible verse, and their favorite Gospel song which would be on file.

Besides Lynne, Margaret, and me, three people signed up on February 1, 2015, one on February 9, 2015, and another on February 15. See, two people were also members of a church in Nelsonville and were reluctant at first to sign but later believed it was fine to do so. I called these people the "founders" of the church, especially Margaret. The church grew more with them and with outside people attending. Prior to COVID-19 we were averaging close to 30 people each Sunday and others, who were unable to attend, I visited on Mondays.

Margaret passed away on Wednesday, February 14, 2018, at the facility. On February 25, the Romans Road Church in the activity room held a Celebration of Life for her. Over 120 people attended. The activities director had to call in an order to rent more chairs to bring in for the service. The Romans Road Church and Devotions with Lynne halted ministry through COVID-19.

At the end of each service, I use Romans 8:28 to witness salvation along with several Scriptures from Romans, especially Romans 8:9-10. This ministry has also produced volunteerism by the residents: Bonnie Clendenin sets up the tables and chairs for services each week; another assists with passing out and collecting songs sheets; an outside volunteer, whose mother was a resident, assists with Communion and song sheets, and others sing or play instruments.

Dale Ellis
Volunteer Ministry to the Lonely
Written by the author after interviewing Mr. Ellis

What can a person who is blind offer to nursing home residents? Dale Ellis with his white cane navigates his way through 111 rooms and suites (not all in one visit) to bring comfort and conversation to those who need human interaction from the outside and who might not have family.

Dale takes the local transportation service two or three times a week to be of aid to residents.

He does more in volunteering in a week than most people might do a lifetime. "What I do," he says, "is find some people who usually don't have visitors. I appreciate all people and want to see them doing well, particularly those who might be lonely. Blind from birth, he's 27 years-old, graduated from high school, went to public schools along the way, and attended a school for the blind for seven years, living on the campus. "They treated me well and I was accepted for who I am."

Dale is now a greeter at a local restaurant and has worked there for seven years. "I want to make a difference to people," he says happily, "because I care about them and their families." He started volunteering nine years ago and he's been very well received. "I went through the volunteer process and trainings. "Most rewarding is letting people know I care and sometimes they look for me. My blessing is knowing that I've made a difference." He says from what he's seen, everybody at the facility is positive and never negative. "They are very polite."

When I think of Dale, I am reminded that no matter what the difficulty or the ability, your life will be enriched by helping others. "Blessing others," he adds, "gives you strength. And when you think you can't go on, my advice is to volunteer in a facility or a hospital and you will discover how blessed you are. Plus, I love the food – the hot dogs during cookouts and the fellowship."

Dale concluded that he volunteers because "helping others, I help myself by boosting my mental and physical health with regular connections; making new friends and building relationships; being in the right place at the right time if there is a job opening; and engaging in exercises that help my memory, functions, and critical thinking."

We should have more Dales in this world.

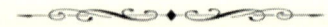

Chapter 10 – Long-Term Care and Social Services: The Glue to Keeping Things Official

Long term care is an increasingly important and rapidly changing component of today's social services delivery system. The need for such services is expected to increase dramatically in the United States as the population ages. Changing demographics have continued to affect the demand for long-term care services and the availability of social workers to provide care to the most vulnerable members of our society, says the National Association of Social Workers (NASW). As the number of individuals in need of long-term care services rises, new issues surrounding staffing, family involvement, quality of life, the role of spirituality, end-of-life care, medical management, program development, and overall service delivery are emerging. The principal components of social work services in long-term care settings are designed to provide assessment, treatment, rehabilitation, and supportive care, and to preserve and enhance social functioning (socialworkers.org).

Service provision requires a unique combination of physical, psychological, and social interventions and family support in order to promote an optimal level of psychological, physical, and social functioning. There have been significant changes in the manner in which appropriate services are delivered across the long-term care spectrum. These services and programs have evolved into a variety of institutional and noninstitutional modalities – the way something exists, is experienced, or expressed. Because the need for them encompasses a wide array of services, many definitions of long-term care exist. Though the need most often arises among older people, some people need long-term care because of physical, mental, or developmental limitations that occur at birth or at any point across the life span.

Whenever you need help, a visit from a family member, counseling, official paperwork, or anything legal, Social Services is the office. Rather unassuming, the myriad tasks they accomplish are incredible. Keeping up with the mental, physical, family, social, well-being, and financial status of the residents is enough in itself. A social worker helps the person entering a new facility make the transition from a previous living environment to life in an institutional setting while meeting that person's comfort needs. Once the resident is established, the social worker assures continuous needs are met and that the resident (and/or the family) is given the opportunity to participate in planning for continual care in the facility, transfer, or discharge back into the community. Although the resident is the main focus, much of the social worker's time might be spent with the family. The resident interacts with all levels of staff.

Long-term care can be provided in a person's own home, in the community, or in a facility. However, even with changing patterns of care, care facilities, as temporary or permanent providers, are still major havens for those who receive social work services in this country. In 1981 the NASW developed Standards for Social Work Services in Long-Term Care Facilities (sociaworkers.org) that are the initial effort to standardize this continually evolving area. It is essential that standards promote sound social work practice and they have been revised to meet changing practices and policies. The standards are a basic social work tool in long-term care facilities, although priorities may vary among settings. The NASW recognizes that knowledge of long-term care services needs to be integrated into social work practice.

Chapter 11 – Bingo! and Its Dynamics: An Activities Necessity

I observed Bingo – judgmentally and critically – without playing for a couple of years. To me, it was an "old person's game." I learned that it's more than a game. It's an institution. Bingo is a major player in nursing home life. Some residents have lost homes, precious possessions, friends, and family members, but Bingo allows residents to say, "The board is mine, the chips, the table space on which I play, and the people with whom I play are mine." It's territorial because often it is all they have – a form of power – lost unwillingly when they had to leave everything and seek care in a nursing home.

Residents bristle over a new activity that might replace Bingo. Nothing doing! They might accept Pokeno every now and then. When Bingo is called, the activity room is full. Not so much so with Pokeno.

Sitting with friends is crucial. I didn't play for a long time but just observed. Following a previous activity, I was still seated with the intention to move before Bingo started. A resident rudely told me, "That's Bonnie's place!" I nodded, smiled, and quickly moved. Changing the playing time is disruptive and confuses the residents. Bingo players don't like change. They want to start on time, play quickly, and keep the room quiet. Interrupting conversation and ringing phones are not acceptable.

"I'm not a Bingo player," I said many times when asked if I was going to play. Guess who has her own cards now and only likes the green chips? Me! I don't play every day and, yes, I like a certain table and playing with certain people. Like everyone else, I now enjoy winning a game or two and leaving with a prize. It's a serious matter, this Bingo.

I read about a Bingo game at a long-term care facility in Canada that evolved into a brawl forcing police to respond. The kerfuffle started with a disagreement between two women – one 79 years old and the other 86 – over a chair. The two women claimed the same seat and neither would give in. The ado turned physical and soon others joined in. Picture it! Canes swinging, wheelchairs swirling, and walkers banging. No one was badly hurt and no arrests were made, but the police said it was quite an unusual call. Whether or not the residents ever got to play Bingo that day is not known.

An aide said to me, "When I catch them playing Bingo, and I am bringing a resident down, I will scream 'Bingo' while they are playing." I said, 'That's a no-no.' The aide continued. 'Oh, yes, but it was always funny. They knew who it was because I did it so often. The players would get upset initially then, toward the end, they would just say, 'Oh, that's her. She is at it again.'" – Aide M.

Bingo is a popular game that can be played for cash and prizes. Bingo is won when a player matches numbers on the card with numbers randomly drawn by a caller. The first person to complete a pattern yells, "Bingo!" Their numbers are checked and a prize or cash awarded. The patterns are varied throughout a gaming session, which keeps players interested and engaged. Bingo is still one of the most popular games and forms of gambling played today.

Bingo is easy to operate with just a couple of staff or volunteers and residents can play along with their visitors. The opportunity to win a small prize or even money is a lure. Its popularity may wane once the elderly population who enjoyed church Bingo in their youth pass on and new generations raised on video games move in.

Side Bar: An aide said the funniest Bingo issue was when the fire alarm went off. The aide told the Bingo players they had to leave the room. That was scarier than someone yelling Bingo! in the middle of a game as a joke. Everyone said, "We are not leaving." The aide said, "It's a fire drill. We <u>have</u> to

*go." The residents said, "No. We are not leaving our cards. "
The aide said, "Okay. Take your cards with you." Case closed.*

Bingo – A Cultural and Generational Experience
*By Tara Winner, April 21, 2014
Cataloger at The Strong National Museum of Play*

Some of my fondest childhood memories date back to the 1970s and '80s when my grandparents would take my sister and me to Friday night Bingo at the local fire hall. The moment we stepped into the building, we were enveloped by the sights, sounds, and aromas of Bingo. Hot dogs, popcorn, and other refreshments were served, and lines formed to purchase the requisite Bingo cards. Often, we sat with my grandparents' "Bingo buddies" at long tables lined with metal folding chairs.

Usually, my sister and I purchased about four heavy, card stock boards and a small handful of "specials." Once seated at the table, our grandmother would pull items out of her Bingo bag and set up our area. She gave us pennies for the "free space," plastic chips for the cards, and daubers (markers used to cover the numbers as they are called) for the specials. Then she'd pull at least 10 to 15 good luck charms out of her bag, each with special meaning for her, although the carved elephants were her favorite. We assembled the trinkets at the top of each board and tickled our fingers across the tops of them for good luck, a familiar routine for many players.

Excitement peaked when someone from our table won. It was customary for the winner to pass the prize money around for everyone to touch, another ritual for good luck. My grand-parents always maintained five times the amount of cards that we kids had, and they would still manage to find numbers on our boards that we missed. For my sister and me, this wasn't just Friday night Bingo – it was an entire cultural experience, and we loved every minute of it.

While researching in The Strong's Brian Sutton-Smith Library and Archives of Play, I learned that Bingo is a derivation of the game Lotto. According to Merilyn Simonds Mohr's book, The New Games Treasury, Lotto, a game of chance, can be traced back to 1530 in Italy where it was known as Lo Giuoco del Lotto de Italia. Unlike Bingo boards, Lotto boards are rectangular with nine squares across and three squares down for a total of 27 squares per board. By the 19th Century, Lotto had spread throughout Europe. Spin-off versions stylized with words and pictures were marketed and sold as educational games.

Bingo was popularized in the United States due to the ingenuity of Edwin S. Lowe. In 1929, the traveling New York salesman spotted a carnival as he passed through Georgia. There he noticed a crowded booth where people were playing a game with hand-stamped boards and beans. He learned that the game was called "Beano," and that the game operator had derived the activity from a Lotto game he had played in Europe. Back in New York, Lowe experimented with numerical combinations on the Beano boards and invited his friends to test out the game. As the legend goes, one of his guests mistakenly called out "Bingo" instead of "Beano" after a winning combination of numbers and the new name stuck.

Lowe began manufacturing Bingo boards in the early 1930s and hired a retired mathematician to devise more than 6,000 different numeric combinations for the boards. Bingo developed wide popularity and churches and fraternal organizations purchased sets to use as fundraisers. At the same time, home versions of the game proliferated and, by the late 1930s, several other companies produced Bingo sets.

Bingo remains popular to this day; in many locations it has even been updated to include electronic boards for players. Home versions of Bingo are still staples of families that have young children. The Strong Museum has more than 20 different versions of Bingo in its collection, including a Superman version. The Brian Sutton-Smith Library and Archives of Play has more than 50 trade catalogs which offer Bingo sets. It all makes me think that I'm well overdue for playing a couple of boards. I may just go back to that fire hall some Friday night, pull out all my good luck charms, and see if I get the chance to yell out "BINGO!" (museumofplay.org)

Chapter 12 – Therapy Dogs: Comfort, Care, and Consolation

Animals play a significant role in healing and in the therapeutic environment. In the 1800s, the idea of Animal Assisted Therapy (AAT) was explored by Florence Nightingale, but it wasn't until 1976 that registered nurse Elaine Smith initiated training for dogs to visit institutions. Today, therapy dogs are used in nursing homes, hospitals, retirement homes, libraries, disaster areas, traumatizing situations, and schools. Some professors take therapy dogs to class to lower students' stress levels and anxiety, temper moods, provide relaxation, and help depression and social skills.

Truly an Angel
Story based on the author's observations

I had a difficult time deciding if I should place Angel among the volunteers or therapy dogs. She is in between because she was, indeed, both. Angel "Nelson" was a special volunteer at a facility in Athens, Ohio. She had her own volunteer badge, along with the tags, around her neck. She was quiet and unassuming – never growling.

Angel was an 11-year-old mixed Boxer Labrador. When her owner Bobbi Nelson, assistant director of activities, moved about, Angel always followed unless she was sunning or dozing by the door. Whether walking quietly and seamlessly between tables at Bingo and other activities, enjoying the sun rays while stretched out at the window, or visiting guests in their rooms, Angel knew her role as a volunteer and as a therapy animal. Residents with arthritic hands straightened them a bit to pet her; those who were pleasantly confused enjoyed her company. Angel sensed when she was needed and went directly to that resident. She was never out of sorts, volunteered with perfection, and was extremely well-trained and behaved. I never heard her bark. If a patient was seriously ill, she would lie close by and provide comfort. Unfortunately, Angel passed away in a house fire. Although she will be sorely missed, her spirit lives on.

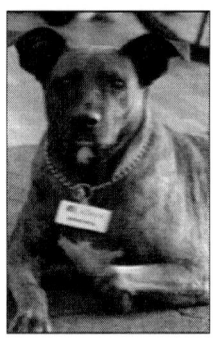

Angel "Nelson"
2009 – August 19, 2020

Canine Care: Therapy dog program launches at O'Bleness Hospital

"I definitely would say that dogs can help with medical care on occasion and can help a lot of patients in some unique ways."
– Steve Trotta

OhioHealth O'Bleness Hospital in Athens has launched a new service for select hospital inpatients. Halle, a 6½ year-old golden retriever is now a certified therapy dog for O'Bleness Hospital. Working alongside her owner, Steve Trotta, a semi-retired physical therapist in the Rehabilitation Department at OhioHealth O'Bleness Hospital, Halle has been making rounds on the third floor of the hospital and visiting with patients who wish to see her during scheduled visiting times. Certified by the stringent standards of Alliance Therapy Dogs, Halle is a fully licensed therapy animal and also meets criteria and standards set forth by OhioHealth. She is considered a volunteer of the hospital. Trotta started Halle's training several years ago. "When I had my first Golden Retriever, several years back, we would often make trips to the Carleton School and Meigs Industries, and I saw the impact it had on adults and students," Trotta said. "I saw that I could continue that with Halle and started bringing her to the PT program at Ohio University. I definitely would say that dogs can help with medical care on occasion and can help a lot of patients in some unique ways." Animal-assisted therapy can impact both the mental and physical sides of recovery healing. Studies from the American Heart Association show decreases in patient anxiety index scores and stress-related hormones after even a brief time is spent with a licensed therapy dog. Halle is the first dog to work in an OhioHealth facility. Wesley, an Australian Labradoodle joined the staff of Riverside Methodist Hospital (Columbus, Ohio) in August of 2017. Following the early success with Halle, O'Bleness plans to expand its program with another therapy dog.

From an OhioHealth news release
In the *Athens News*, March 25, 2019

Steve Trotta
Therapy Animals (in his own voice)

Early in my career as a physical therapist, we had our first golden retriever, Quincy. I took him to a nursing home and when I went by myself that was the most important part.

The lady wouldn't see me unless I had him along. This time I had Quincy with me.

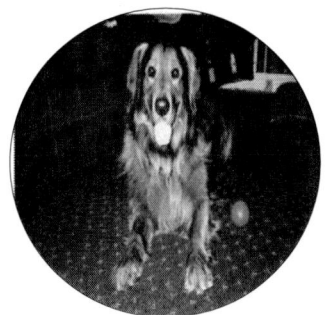

Quincy

There's something about animals, especially dogs, that makes a difference. It is quite rewarding for the patients when the dogs just curl up on the patient. I really appreciate it when they allow the animals to do that. It makes a difference for there is something about dogs and other animals in facilities that help people. That was the most important part about the first facility I visited. The dog curled up on a patient and something clicked in with me after that and I always brought Quincy when I could. That's why we have Halle now. It's been rewarding and takes patience. She's really good with sad situations, with staff, and with students.

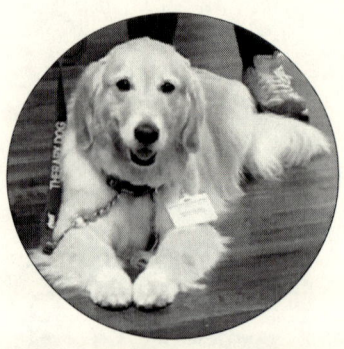

Halle

Halle visits mostly at hospitals, but a resident at a local facility saw her and asked for Halle to come to her room because she once had a golden retriever. Halle immediately went to her as the resident patted her knee for her to come. Therapy dogs provide stress relief for physical therapy, anatomy students, and other students. I take her to my classroom or lab frequently.

Chapter 13 – Abuse: A Student's Perspective

"Nursing home abuse should never happen, and yet it's more common than you may think. It causes devastation in families – to see people they love suffer from types of abuse that are just unacceptable. Knowledge is the first step in preventing nursing home abuse. Be sure to choose a nursing home carefully."

Elder abuse is a huge problem in the United States and something needs to be done about it! The effect on the elderly is catastrophic. According to an article published in 2018 by the World Health Organization (WHO, who.int) elderly individuals who are abused are two times more likely to die prematurely than those who are not. Hospitalization is also more likely to occur if the individual had been abused. Abuse puts a major physiological strain on the elderly person which can lead to depression, fear, anxiety, and even suicide.

Abuse in nursing homes is unlawful, demeaning, and happens all too often. Imagine living in a nursing home, and being called names, yelled at, ignored, and even beaten. This seems unlikely. Right? Wrong. It happens way more than you think. According to the Nursing Home Abuse Center (CNHA, nursinghomeabusecenter.com) one to two million elder Americans are abused by caregivers each year. Maybe you have a parent or grandparent living in a nursing home or, like me, you work in one. Insensitivity by caregivers, lack of training, lack of reporting, and rare consequences are all reasons for recurring abuse.

Abuse isn't just physical, it can be categorized as emotional, financial, neglect, and even sexual. The CNHA reports the loss of 2.9 billion dollars per year can be linked to financial abuse.

Statistics show just how bad elder abuse is. The WHO says two to three employees at an undisclosed nursing home admitted to some form of abuse of residents. The CNHA reports about 6.3 million people older than 85 years old were abused in 2010; the number is projected to increase to 17.9 million by the year 2050. The Center explains that seven to 10% of individuals over the age of 65 suffered from abuse in 2016 alone. Elder abuse, however, isn't confined just to health care professionals. Ninety percent of all elder abuse is committed by a family member. This chance is increased if drugs and alcohol factor into the equation.

Financial abuse is categorized as theft of money or property, over-charging by a nursing home, charging a higher co-pay, and more. The CNHA asserts that financial exploitation occurs at a rate of 41 out of every 1,000 individuals surveyed. Dementia puts people at a higher risk of abuse because they often do not remember the events and the abuser can get away with abuse much easier. In addition, 5.1 million elderly people in the U.S. have some form of dementia. Forty-seven percent of patients with dementia suffered from some kind of abuse, according to the National Center for Victims of Crime (victims ofcrime.org). The complaint breakdown is 27.4% is physical abuse, 22.1% is resident-on-resident abuse, 19.4% is psychological abuse, 15.3% is gross neglect, 7.9% is sexual abuse and, lastly, 7.9% is financial exploitation. Men and women are both victims of elder abuse, but two out of every three elder abuse victims are women.

Although the data might be surprising, it is believed that these statistics are very much higher since elderly abuse goes undocumented. The elderly fear the abuser and retaliation. They may not remember the encounter or are physically unable to report it due to other disabling limiting factors.

A National Public Radio (npr.org) article written in 2017 by Ian Jaffe describes a detective who uncovered 134 cases of elder abuse that sent residents to the hospital. These incidents were simply swept under the rug and the detective is quoted as saying, "A woman was left deeply bruised after being sexually assaulted at her nursing home. Not following federal law, the nursing home never reported the incident. They cleaned off the victim. In doing so, they destroyed all of the evidence that law enforcement could have used as part of the investigation into this crime. They even went so far as to contact the local police department to say they did not need to come out to the facility and investigate."

The Organization for Nursing Home Abuse Justice (nursinghomeabuse.org) estimates in 2019 that only one in 14 occurrences of elder abuse is formally reported. When it comes to abuse from a family member which, again, accounts for 90% of all elder abuse cases, many of these cases aren't reported because the elderly are afraid to see their family member get in trouble or the person believes they deserve it because they feel like a burden needing help with daily activities of life.

Elderly people need your assistance and here's what you can do to help stop this growing problem. Look for the signs of elder abuse including bruising, scratches, skin tears, pressure sores, a decreased mental state not related to the medical diagnoses, and anything that seems out of the ordinary. If you suspect that your loved one is being abused, call the facility's ombudsman – the number would be posted in the nursing home – or call the state's ombudsman to report the issue(s) and get your loved one transferred to a better long-term care facility with a higher amount of qualified staff.

Nursing home abuse should never happen, and yet it's more common than you may think. It devastates families – to see people they love suffer from abuse that is just unacceptable. Knowledge is the first step in preventing nursing home abuse. Be sure to choose a nursing home carefully.

According to the Organization for Nursing Home Abuse Justice's article published in 2019, some other ways the elderly can avoid abuse and get help are: Use a living will; maintain a strong social life; get involved in the community and in the activities of the facility; manage their own finances, if possible, to avoid financial abuse; keep a personal phone and know who to call when help is needed; report all abuse to the adult protective services; file a police report; and keep a hidden record of all instances of abuse.

You can do your part to give the elderly the retirement life they deserve by educating yourself as well as anyone else in contact with the elderly about the horror of elder abuse. Imagine if it was someone you love lying in a bed in a nursing home being abused and neglected. You would be infuriated. I've seen in my job as an STNA that not everyone in these long-term care facilities have family members to visit them. Who is going to advocate on their behalf? You can! If you follow some of the simple steps that I have covered, you can help people who so desperately need it.

By Michael Scott
STNA and Nursing Student

Side Bar: A number of online resources provide a state-by-state summary of nursing home laws. The Nursing Home Abuse Center was founded to bring justice to those affected by nursing home and elder abuse. Their mission is to educate and empower victims of abuse and their families to take a stand against this unlawful mistreatment. They work to return dignity back to those who have been broken down by nursing home abuse and neglect (nursinghomeabusecenter.org).

Stories of Love and Loss

What follows are personal stories.
These are first and second-hand
accounts of people's experiences.
Their stories are edited for length and clarity.

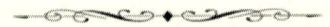

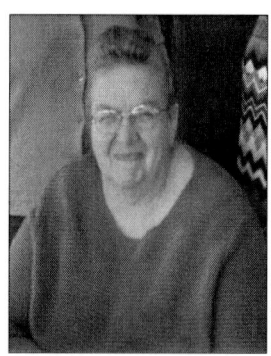

Margaret Dalene Baker

Chapter 14 – Margaret Dalene Baker

Spiritual Compass
Written by the author after interviewing
Margaret Dalene Baker

"Because of really bad arthritis,
I can hardly walk or go to the bathroom by myself."

Dalene is from Logan, Ohio. She attended high school there and worked at a convenience store for 23 years. She had to enter long-term skilled care because of really bad arthritis and because she can hardly walk or go to the bathroom by herself.

"You won't believe it, but I was a very shy person and was not very outgoing. Once I started working, I came out of shyness," stated Dalene. Her dad wasn't like that. He could talk to anybody. "Now, I like to meet new people and like showing people crafts. I try to show my good side all the time.

I might not be in a good mood all the time, but I like to show good to other people. There's a few in here that are not like that." Dalene now loves to meet people and although she hasn't traveled much – Maryland and North Carolina – she is well read and knowledgeable. She has three sisters and a brother. Two sisters live in Logan who provide a strong support system and one lives in North Carolina. Her brother passed away. Her parents took her to church when she was just four. Dalene recounted her story:

"Yes, I went to church my whole life and my parents went to church their whole lives, too. I was a Sunday school teacher for about 30 years and sang in the choir, but I don't sing solos. My great-grandmother went to church, but I never got to meet her because I was only one year-old when she died. Pentecostal is my denomination.

"Pastor Ivan came here to this facility and his wife said it was really a nice place. I didn't like the facility where I lived and my sister inquired. That's why I'm here. I would like to go home one day but I'm still needing help with my showers and I have to be cautious with standing. I can get out of bed and keep my mind strong by coloring and crocheting. I have more use of my fingers now by going through therapy. I frame my pictures and hang some on the wall and get involved in activities. Now, when I first came here, I stayed in my room for two or three months because I didn't want to be here. I didn't want to be bothered until I went up the hallway one day and someone invited me to eat with them in the dining room. I started from there and now they can't find me in my room (she laughs).

"I've got heart issues and I've got an ulcer. My mobility is not great as I have arthritis in my knees and shoulders, but they're getting better through therapy. I am doing occupational therapy and not physical therapy now. My family is really supportive. They used to come every day but now that I'm getting better, she comes once a week. My sister is very supportive of me.

"I'm surprised at the love here. When I first came the staff started getting used to you and would say I love you. I'm not used to that and I thought, okay. The nurses and even the housekeepers learn your names and they talk to you. They are very supportive of church services and things like that. This is important to me and I love meeting new people. There are a few people in here that don't get along with each other. I told the activities director, that it puts me in the middle because I try to be friendly with everybody."

Her favorite food is fruit. Since she has been here, she has gained friends and a stable environment. "There are a lot of people who will help," she said. She lost being able to drive and her independence. "I had a hard time letting people help me, I always did things for myself. Now if I need help, I ask for it."

She has no other losses as she rented where she lived and did not own a home. Most of her things are in storage. Her brother was in a nursing home for three years. What she has found different from other places is, "Here there are spiritual things and therapy here is really good. You think, 'All they are doing is pushing me.' If they hadn't pushed me, I wouldn't be where I am at now. And yes, you have certain favorites. Losing physical capacity is upsetting. It upsets me when I know I can do something, but I'm limited now. You just have to work with what you've got. This is the way I am and I just have to go with it."

"Study to show thyself approved unto God,
a workman that needed not to be
ashamed, rightly dividing the Word of truth."
– II Timothy 2:15

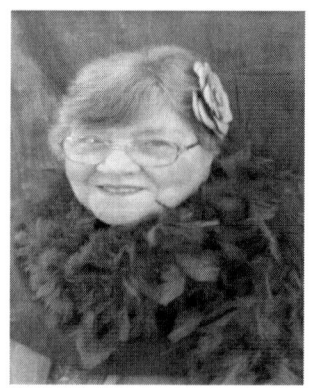

Alma Spencer

Chapter 15 – Bobbi Nelson (Alma Spencer)

A Daughter's Delight
Bobbi Nelson's recollections of her mother, Alma Spencer

"My support as a family member was important to her.
I was here every day. I helped with activities and all which,
in turn, got me a job in activities."

My mom, Alma Spencer, was born April 20, 1932. At the end of her life she resided in a facility for about four years. Before that, I took care of her at home for five years. My mom was paralyzed from the chest down from back surgery gone wrong. She had a tumor embedded in her spinal cord that pinched off the cord and damaged it to the extent it could not be repaired. Her paralysis affected her bowels and bladder, so she had an ostomy (an opening in the abdomen allowing waste to exit the body). She had catheters, bedsores, and a lot of other health conditions. She was also diabetic. There were just a variety of health conditions.

She was an amazingly strong woman. Now is when I will cry because my mom taught me that no matter what happens, you can get through it. I'll never forget her moving a dresser by herself and I got mad at her because she said it was easy. She just put a rug under the dresser and slid it. She said, "Where there's a will, there's a way," and that was my mom's motto. As long as you can figure out a way to do it, it could be done. She lived to be 84 years-old and, even after the surgery, she was an amazing lady. She was positive and I will always admire her for that.

She was a factory worker. She retired then went back to work because she didn't like being retired. She was an activities assistant, so I'm following in her footsteps. She worked at a local nursing home in Morgan County and loved being around the people and making them smile. My mom didn't lose any mental capacity, but she lost mobility. It was very hard because on a Monday she worked an eight-hour shift. On Tuesday, she had back surgery and she came out of it paralyzed. I quit my job and moved in with her. It was a major, major lifestyle change for all of us, our entire family, but she kept her spirits up and she always thought that she would walk again. She was always positive about that and would try as long as therapy would work with her. I saw her stand a few times but, as for walking, she never achieved that.

I was her primary caregiver. We had a lot of trouble finding dependable and knowledgeable home health care workers to come in and help. People would be very enthusiastic about helping, but they didn't know what they were doing. I actually had one lady drop mom on the toilet and break open the wound that we had been working on for months to heal. I'll never forget all of the blood. When the worker released the Hoyer lift to put mom down on the toilet, she just flipped the lever instead of releasing it gradually and mom dropped onto the toilet. So that was, you know, the home health care and with the insurance and the transportation, we had a lot of issues.

We were well-known in Morgan County because I would load my mom in the truck, put the Hoyer lift and the wheelchair in the bed of the truck and down the road we would go to the grocery store. We would go wherever we needed to go. And I thank God for that – I really don't know how I did it because I have a bad back myself, but I did it and I'm so happy that I was able to take care of my mother.

I miss her so much. She was my best friend. Excuse me (Bobbi cries). I could tell my mom anything and she was never judgmental. She always said, "It'll be all right, honey." She was a positive lady. From her background, she never knew her mother Her dad was abusive. Her mother was so strong to put up with him for 32 years until the kids were grown. I really love my mother and I can't wait to see her again.

At the facility, my support as a family member was important to her. I was there every day. I helped with activities and all which, in turn, got me a job, but I volunteered a lot before I started working. I just had to see my mom every day and we talked on the phone numerous times a day. She was a resident, you know, and things happened that she needed to tell me about. I tried to always be there for my mama.

We have residents who don't have family support and individuals who don't have very much family. They don't come around as often as I feel they should. I think they've given up and act like their family member has already passed, especially if they've lost their memory. I bought some twinkling Christmas lights and put them in an individual's room so she could lie in bed and watch them. So, you know, I try to do stuff to help everybody because I am so fortunate that I was able to be there for my mom and help her through all of this.

As I mentioned, my mom was at another nursing home before. I actually took her out because she laid in urine and she had to share a room. The bathroom doorways were not even big enough for a wheelchair to pass through. It was horrible. I went in one day and when I saw her lying in urine, I went right out and told the nurse, "I'm taking her home." They told me I couldn't and that's when I said, "Watch me." So, I took my mother home and that's how I ended up taking care of her at home for so long. Then my daughter started working in this nursing home and told us what a nice place this is. We came over for a visit to give mom a tour. We got her put on the waiting list to be a resident. So, it all worked out.

She liked to play cards. Euchre. She used to play this double-handed Euchre which used two decks of cards. I couldn't keep track of what was going on and she would just laugh at me because she loved to play cards. She also loved Bingo. I'll never forget the day my daughter and I were visiting her in her room, but when it was Bingo time, she up and left. My daughter and I were sitting there like, "Okay, I guess we'll leave, too." People here don't realize Bingo serves several purposes: socialization, hand/eye/dexterity coordination, and thinking.

(Burst of laughter) The funniest story I can think of is after my mom was paralyzed, she was reclining in her chair and had her blankie and everything. My daughter and I and a couple of Mom's friends, and our dogs, were in the room and one of the dogs farted. It was a unique smell that no one wanted to stick around and endure. So, we all jumped up and ran out of the room and, I'm sorry, but I'm going to tell you exactly word for word what my mother said, "You sons of b_ _ _ _ _ _. I'll come back and haunt you." She couldn't get out of her chair. She couldn't move. I had to get rid of my dogs when mom got ill because I couldn't take care of them. I raised German Shepherds for years, but I couldn't do everything. Mom was the most important.

I wish I had spent more time with her before she got hurt. Before the surgery, I would call her when I was coming home from work and tell her to put a pot of coffee on and I could always remember the thrill in her voice because she was so glad that I was going to spend time with her. It kind of makes me feel bad that I wasn't there more. So, I hope and I pray that my kids will be the same with me if I get in a situation like my mother. I think my kids would do the same for me.

It's still all fresh, though it's been a few years since she passed, but my life has moved on. I met someone that I didn't have time to be with before because taking care of mom was a 24/7 job. Actually, I met a man in mom's facility. His wife was ill and she passed about the same time that mom did. We went through the group grieving process together and we have since developed a really nice relationship. We went to Florida on vacation. So, yeah, I have moved on. I'll never forget my mother, but she would want me to be happy. There is a song that every time I hear it on the radio, I have to pull over because I'm crying so bad. It's Rascal Flatts' "I Won't Let Go." It suits me and mom because that was us. I'm not, I'm not going to let go of her.

It's kind of a coincidence that my mother died on December 3 because my fiancé died on December 3. For my mom and my fiancé to die on the same day, 30 years apart was hard, very hard. I think mom did that on purpose so I'd only have one day to mourn.

I was raised on a hog farm. My mother and father had about 120 female hogs that had babies twice a year. I didn't have many friends because I always smelled like a hog, but it taught me the value of working and to not give up. You have to work for what you want. You (Dr. Lewis) remind me a lot of my mother. Your smile and your love for life. Your faith and your situation remind me so much of my mother. You're very similar and I just love your smile. I love the attitude that you're always positive, like she was. Mom was the president of Resident Council at the facility and she was very motivational. You are, too.

I feel that a lot of people here need that motivation and they need someone to stand back and clap when they're in therapy working on something. They need that. They need someone to know that somebody noticed what they did and their hard work because a lot of them just give up. It's so hard to get from point A to point B that they just don't even try anymore."

"And now abideth faith, hope, love, these three, but the greatest of these is love." – I Corinthians 13:13

Alma passed December 3, 2016

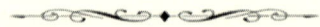

Chapter 16 – A Daughter's Dilemma

Relative relating her story prefers to remain anonymous

*"She's lonely. She feels like while there are
some really good aides, people are
way too busy. Things are not done right.
When she puts a buzzer on, she waits forever.
She's always hated the food. She's just a fussy eater."*

My mother graduated from high school and was a homemaker, what she calls "a domestic engineer." Born in 1922, she worked in a factory for a short period of time. She traveled every summer to Pennsylvania because of my father's family which was from there. My mother's travels included Las Vegas, Hawaii, and California. She and my father had four children. Two had Muscular Dystrophy and one died in 1979 and the other died in 1980. My father died in 1985 and my mother then lived by herself in Lorain, Ohio. When I moved to Athens, she moved to be close to me and her grandchildren.

My mother had been at a different facility for a couple years and then another one, which offered assisted living, opened and she just kind of needed a change. It was a newer site and was beautiful. We made the decision and she was one of the first people there – six months before anybody else came. They weren't allowed to take more people as it was a test. My mother's main issue was really bad arthritis, osteoarthritis. She also had the atrial fibrillation, irregular heartbeat, and then she broke her femur which was a big to-do.

She's lonely. She feels like while there are some really good aides, people are way too busy. Things are not done right. When she puts a buzzer on, she waits forever. She's just a fussy eater and she has always hated the food and the often impersonal care. There's a lot of turnover in terms of things. People will say they'll come back then they don't. You know, there are some kind people, but there are people who don't know how to lift her, so they hurt her. She's very fragile. Just since Christmas, they've lost her dentures and they lost her hearing aids, and it's no small fee to get new dentures at her age or to get new hearing aids. It's taken three months to get the hearing aids.

The response of the facility, in my opinion, is often slower than desired. With the teeth, they did get right on it to try to replace them and they did pay for the new teeth. But, in the meantime, it took a long time to get the teeth and the follow through and watching her are poor. They would give her food she couldn't chew so then they ordered a soft diet. The next day, they brought her a whole piece of pizza – she has no teeth! On the surface it looks like there's a response because I'm sure their records say a soft diet was ordered, but then it was not delivered.

They were bringing her hard crackers for a snack and I'm honestly just waiting to see if anybody ever figures it out. It looks like they brought her plain yogurt. My mother does not like plain yogurt. So, day after day after day, she's not eating it. I go there and I get her something else that she likes. Lots of times there's no spoon. You have a cup of yogurt but no spoon. Or, they leave her snack so she could kind of start to chew the crackers, except nobody opens them for her. She can't open them.

I think they need to be more attentive. There needs to be better communication. Some of the aides are just worn out. It's a rough job and they need more people to make sure they're providing the care that's advertised. I would say the physical therapy is very good. I'm very happy with physical therapy.

She has great family support – her grandchildren, my husband and me, and my older sister. My mother has always been about family and if my kids call her, it just makes her day. When they come home, she loves it.

A really funny story that we laugh about still was when my sister got married. She was 10 years older than me and I was 13. Our church was a mile from our house and my mom was a nervous wreck because she had to drive my sister to the church. My brothers were in wheelchairs and disabled. My father had to go get them, take them to church, and get them all settled in. My mom didn't act like the mother of the bride. She worked herself up about having to literally drive a mile to the church. We're in our driveway and all of the neighbors were out watching because there's the bride and she's here in the driveway. My aunt is behind her with the bridal party and I'm with my aunt and my mother is so nervous. Now, this is the main event. My mom forgot to look behind her and she rammed right into my aunt's car. We laughed about that for years.

We've had lots of fun, lots of good times. Mom liked to read which is increasingly hard for her. She loves cooking and baking and was a really good cook. Putting her hands in dough was like therapy. We all got cooking from her.

With overall care, the problem is the system is broken. Right? It's easy to blame the individuals because they're on the front line, but it's the bigger system that's broken in terms of just nursing home care generally. Most of these are for-profit places, so they try to maximize their profit and the care is not what it should be. Aides need more training and need to be paid more. They see residents when no one else does, not even nurses or administration or whomever. I pity the people like my mom – even though she's quite fragile and frail, she's very smart and she's lucid. If some aide comes in and starts grabbing her arm, she says, "Don't grab my arms because I have such bad arthritis." But, you know, you're at their mercy, right? And also, my mom has me looking in and making sure that people are doing what they are supposed to do. But some of these poor people have nobody.

I complain all the time. I come at different times so they don't know when I'll be there. They were loading my mom in the van for a test that they forgot to tell me about and my mom said, "Where's my daughter?" She knows I wouldn't let her go out of the building without me and she said, "You better call my daughter before you put me on this van." So they called me and I said, "No, no, no. She's not going all the way to Lancaster to do a test that I don't believe she needs." Remember, it was my mom who said, "You better call my daughter," and I said to my mom, "Good girl! You do not go out of this building without my knowledge." Not everybody has that, you know, and that's why facilities have to get on the ball. There are not enough people; there are not enough trained people.

When there's a problem, nobody knows anything and that's the other thing that just irks me. It's like, "I don't know." If my mom denies it, they'll say, "Oh, your mom denied it and it didn't happen." If my mom says, "Yes, it happened." They'll assert that my mom's confused to make it always to their advantage. We've got some pretty good aides on this floor now and over the past year there's been about three that we wouldn't allow back in here. Just no. There were two that put her to bed one night and lost her teeth. I know well that they dropped them along the way because teeth don't walk away, Mom can't throw them away, and we were here probably 15 minutes after they put her to bed and they could have been in the garbage can. There were two sisters who were the aides and I said, "You guys are done. No." They were really bad news because there was an incident before when my mom told me one of them was yelling at her. Of course, the aide denied it all.

You have to talk really slowly to my mom. She reads lips a lot and I don't think the physician has a clue my mom can't hear. He's been treating her for two years. The thing that made me really mad is when she broke her femur. Of course, they had her all doped up because she was in a lot of pain and everything. But one day the physician comes. He has his hat and his coat on – doesn't take them off – sits down and he looks up at me and he goes, "Now what medicine did we put her on?" I just looked at him and said, "We didn't put her on anything. You put her on medicine." And I said, "Actually, I have that same question." I am a clinician and I told him before I see my patients I usually go look at their charts. He's the worst and then we get billed every week for like $85 and he doesn't see my mom. Sorry (she cries). This is my mom. He's got a good deal going, right? My mom is billed $85 a week. He doesn't see her. I doubt he's touched my mom and doesn't check vital signs. That's the other thing with some of the nurses, too. They don't take the time to talk to my mom. She can't hear and you just have to slow it down. It's a process. They come in they talk to her and she can't hear a word they're saying.

There are some good people. I told the administrator that the nurses need to have more respect for the aides because they're the backbone here. Make it or break it. I feel that the nurses should be the ones who are really modeling very good behavior and I don't feel that they consistently do.

"And God shall wipe away all tears from their eyes; and there shall be no more death, neither sorrow, nor crying, neither shall there be any more pain; for the former things are passed away."
– Revelation 21:4

Her mother transitioned in 2019.

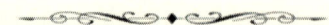

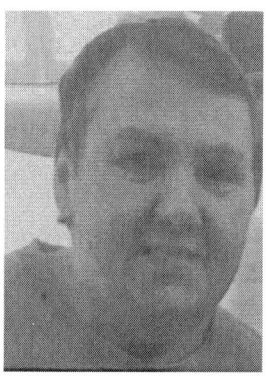

Bonnie Clendenin

Chapter 17 – Bonnie Clendenin

A New Friend
Written by the author after interviewing Bonnie Clendenin

*"My family put me in here because I fell and
could not get up. I tried to stand
and fell back. They came and got me and
they put me in here. I couldn't walk."*

Bonnie was leery of me, my singing in church especially, and very protective of the pastor and the services. I
wondered why she seemed to hate me. She ignored me when
I spoke to her. She vocally opposed my singing in church – not
that I was a bad vocalist. She helped form the church and was
territorial. I thought she was prejudiced, yet she would speak
to my daughter. I made it a point to be kind. Nothing worked
until the pastor opened the door for me to interview her for
this book. She was extremely amiable. Here's what I learned.

I had to remember one of my mottos, "First seek to under-stand."

Bonnie has a hearing problem and didn't hear me most times I spoke to her or hear what I was singing; had a terrible fall that created memory lapses; lost her children; experienced a horrible childhood; has extremely crippling arthritis; and cannot read or write. Understood. Everyone has a backstory.

She said, "I used to go to ATCO (Advocacy, Training, Career, Opportunities) in Athens County and made pens. I have been at this facility a long time. I was married and had two boys. When I got into a bit of trouble, my boys were taken away from me. I have pictures at the house. My husband passed away and my issues are arthritis in my hands and feet which are severely crippled."

That doesn't stop Bonnie. In spite of the serious problem with her feet, Bonnie sets up and arranges tables for church and activities. She likes Bingo and shopping trips, and watches Westerns and Andy Griffin. Her sister visits and her brothers take her to the doctor. She has been in numerous hospitals. The friends she has in the facility and the nurses are important to her. "It's cool that this will be in a book," she said.

Here's what I did: I offered to teach her to read and/or write and engaged her in conversation about those things I had learned she liked; I got closer to her to talk so that she could hear; we shared pizza and other goodies; I gave her any gifts I won at the monthly auction; I acknowledged her birthday, and was genuinely interested in her – loving, nice, and kind. The late great Fred Rogers of PBS' Mister Rogers' Neighborhood said he had three principles in life: "Be kind. Be kind. Be kind."

Bonnie became my new "best" friend. She saved Sunday newspapers for me, made sure I was welcome wherever she was sitting, and always had a smile for me. Through loving kindness, I drew her.

> *"The Lord hath appeared of old unto me, saying,*
> *Yes, I have loved thee with an everlasting love:*
> *therefore with loving kindness have I drawn thee."*
> *– Jeremiah 31:3*

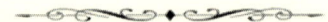

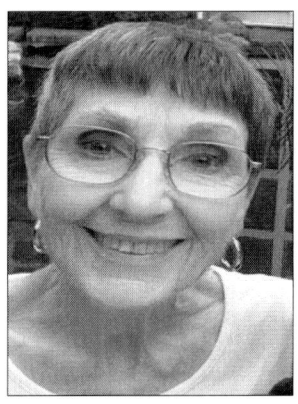

Patricia Morrison

Chapter 18 – Molly Morrison (Patricia Morrison)

In Her Voice
Daughter Molly Morrison speaks through the eyes
and the lived experiences of her mother Trish

"He [Trish's husband] started falling and I started becoming more forgetful. I knew it because it was painful and frightening. I knew that I was forgetting things, too."

My name is Patricia "Trish" Morrison, born December 5, 1933, in a very small town called Shamrock, Texas, and raised in Hedley, Texas, another very, very small town. My father and mother were young when they married. She was 17. They married in Alabama and went to Texas. My father was from Alabama, or that general area, and was a cotton farmer. She was a homemaker and may have finished grade school or junior high. Women didn't have careers at that time. My father never owned any land he farmed. He always worked the land of someone else.

I was number nine of 10 children. My parents got married in 1911 and I was a depression baby. That affected me throughout my life. It showed. I didn't want to throw things away and I was very cautious about things like that. I wasn't close with my mother. My mother and father were very strict and my mother wasn't a very affectionate person. I was very afraid of my father as he was so strict. He could just lash out at you. He would joke, but if he got angry at you, he would just lash out.

We had a good upbringing. We went to church every Sunday. My parents raised us in The Church of Christ and they taught us; we were raised well. All of my siblings and I finished high school and that was a big deal in that era. I had almost finished high school and had a boyfriend named James Potts. He wanted to get married when we finished. I knew that I didn't want to marry him. I knew that would mean a similar type of "never get out of there, never get out of Hedley" life. I was upset about it and one of the few times I confided in my mother, I told her I was very sad about my boyfriend that he had asked me to marry him and I had turned him down, and that he cried. I was sad because it hurt me and, as I told my mother about it, she was unsympathetic. In fact, she laughed, poked fun at him and said, "Oh, ho, ho, ho, I wish I could have seen his long face when you told him." She was very cavalier about it and that hurt my feelings. My mother could often be very hateful and short. She would always make me feel bad and was critical or negative, and now I know she was probably tired. Tired of different places, and having all of those kids, but still she hurt me a lot and I always wished I had a better relationship with my mother right up until the end.

At that point, I thought I was going to try to go to college. I went to Abilene Christian University in Abilene, Texas. Of course, my parents couldn't pay for anything like that, so I went to Seattle, Washington, to live with my sister who was 20 years older than me. She was like a second mother. She was a difficult individual and very bossy but did a lot for me. She made me remember it, too. I went to live with her and I remember my feelings were really hurt by her because I had an accent. I wanted some nail polish and I remember the color was Pink Tinge. I had an accent which was fairly strong, and I called it Pink "Teenge." My sister was critical and told me not to pronounce it like that.

I lived with my sister and her husband and didn't have to pay room and board. My job was with a temporary agency that employed girls for secretarial work. I saved my money and my sister contributed as well for me to go to college. I finished my degree in three-and-a-half years in elementary education and I wish I had had someone more interested in guiding me because I didn't get the best of grades. I think it was because I didn't know how to study and, of course, I wasn't from a family who had gone to college. I did get my degree and I was always very proud of that. I called it my sheepskin.

One summer when I was with my sister and working, there was a man who called for a girl working temporarily in the office. I had to speak with him and he recognized my accent. We got to talking, and he invited me to lunch. He arrived one day at lunch time and I had never actually seen him. He said, "Oh, I thought you were blonde" and that made me mad. I think he expected this petite, blonde, southern belle with an accent. So, I said, "Well, I didn't know you wore glasses either." He was a nice man and I decided to marry him. He had a college degree and was in the armed service but was never shipped out of the States. His brother was killed by a kamikaze plane in World War II.

My husband, George Morrison, worked in the States. He repaired damaged aircraft carriers that were used by fighter pilots in training in the United States before they were used by fighter pilots abroad. He went to college on the GI (Government Issue) Bill and I went to college as well. As I mentioned, my sister paid for a good portion of my education and she never let me forget it. I paid every cent back to her. It took me a while, but I did it. George and I lived in Marysville, Washington, his hometown. I was a first-grade teacher and George was an insurance underwriter. Much later, we went to Portland, Oregon, and I had my daughter Molly there. I had just one child. None of my siblings had more than three or four children and I wonder if that is because we came from such a big family ourselves. I remember when I was small, hearing someone talk about my mother being pregnant again and that would have been with my youngest brother. I was number nine, he was number 10, and my oldest sister was 20 years old. It was not a joyous time and someone said, "Oh, break the news to Blanche gently." That was my oldest sister's name. That was because someone had to tell her that our mother was pregnant again and my sister, with whom I lived, sent my parents word that it was not good having all of these children.

While in Portland, I was a substitute teacher for a while and, later, when Molly was still small, we moved to California and I got a job in the printing business and became the manager. My husband decided he didn't want to do insurance anymore and worked in a home improvement business. We wanted to buy the business and the owner dragged his feet. While I was manager, the business started to thrive and he wouldn't sell it. I was a people person and I really knew how to bring in the people. I bought a printing place across the street and the other owner who wouldn't sell, should have known better. Our business did extremely well and he had to close his business. We fixed it up and had this business for many years, no health problems so far. I had walking partners and we walked a lot, but I was also on my feet for long periods in the business. When you own a business, it owns you. I was always worried about money and we couldn't afford to buy insurance, so we couldn't go to the doctor very much if we did get sick.

We had that business for 20 years. We struggled a lot. After our daughter Molly finished her Ph.D., she traveled a while in Italy then moved to Athens, Ohio, where she got a job as a professor. She didn't want to be far from us and we didn't want to be far from her either, so we closed our business. We didn't sell it because those chain stores came in and would have knocked us out of business anyway. So, we closed our business, sold our house, and moved right next door to Molly in 2001. I got to travel a lot and went to Italy 11 times. Her father got to go on some trips and we would never have been able to go otherwise. She took us to Maine, to Massachusetts, and several times to Philadelphia where we would go and look at museums. We still did quite well with our health, but my husband started becoming very forgetful and he got prostate cancer which was discovered when he went to the doctor. He had successful treatment but, while he was there, the doctor noticed there were some other issues going on and prescribed a medication which my husband didn't want to take. It was very expensive, and we tended to think the doctor's worry at his not taking the pills was hogwash, but the doctor was right. My husband was becoming very forgetful. It was discovered that he had dementia and, at that point, he had to take the medication.

We got along quite well for several years. He wasn't allowed to drive so I would drive us places and he would come along with me. Over the years, it became increasingly difficult because he became unsteady on his feet. I was his primary caregiver, although our daughter sort of cared for both of us. She was there for everything. The main care was by me and he was still very easy. Toward the end, it became more difficult and Molly wound up taking care of both of us. Then my husband got more memory loss and increasingly unstable on his feet. He started falling and I became more forgetful. It was painful and frightening because I knew that I was forgetting things. I knew some things about that because of my husband. My daughter was extremely worried and always stressed out about us. She even had one of her colleagues ride with me while I was driving to see if it was just her thinking I wasn't a good driver anymore or if the colleague thought so, too. The colleague thought I should not be driving, but Molly was hesitant to do anything about it immediately. I can understand. You just can't take away one's driving license and I don't know if I would have listened to her anyway. Luckily, or thankfully, because it did turn out to be a blessing.

A horrible thing happened. Molly worked abroad every summer and worried about us while she was gone. One summer she bought a freezer and put it in our laundry room. She was going to cook enough meals for the entire six-week period she would be gone and put them in the freezer so that I could just pull those out and heat them up. She started working on those slowly in advance. When I went to my exercise class, my husband would wait for me in the lobby. He wasn't a wanderer at that time. Then I started getting really forgetful, too, about where I should pull off on the exit when driving, so I figured it would be okay if I just stopped on the freeway to see where I should turn off. I stopped the car in the center lane and I was violently rear ended. It was a horrible, horrible accident. It tore up our car and we were taken to the emergency room. I called my daughter and my husband had to be taken to Columbus. I had a cut on my head which was stitched up. My husband was in the trauma center and, because of my own increasing forgetfulness, I wasn't able to do anything because I was so upset. My own dementia was coming on rapidly and my daughter had to take family leave from work to take care of us. The doctor told her I had Alzheimer's and the officer said I could not have a license. Luckily the accident didn't kill either of us, but I was not allowed to drive. To keep my dignity, Molly blamed the officer that I couldn't have a license. I told my daughter well, "I guess I'm an old lady now."

I was not fit to do anything. She put a sleeper in her house and my husband would get up and roam around. He tried to urinate in the sink. He got up several times in the night and got combative with my daughter. He locked the doors, screamed and shouted, and wasn't his regular self. She realized she could not take care of him and she could not get him into the rest home because the insurance refused. She tried to get the doctors to help, did all kinds of paperwork, wrote letters, and he was refused over and over again. She realized this couldn't go on and eventually she was referred to a lady at a new facility who helped her and was able to get him a room in March 2015.

The battle had just started then because Molly knew it would be impossible to bring him back home because he needed all sorts of therapy and there was no way she could take care of him and me, too, because he would fall. She was able to take the rest of the semester off because it was a full-time job taking care of both of us. She finally got him on Medicaid and on long-term rather than just temporary care, which was a big load off her mind. Molly and I would go visit him every day and he was eating pretty well. They decided to put him in a wheel-chair because they were afraid he would fall, but he did not like being in that wheelchair. Molly and the people at the facility would devise all kinds of ways to keep him in it. He thought they were mean when they were just trying to help him. He couldn't remember that he was told not to get out of the wheelchair and they would put alarms on his blanket and on the wheelchair and he would do all kinds of things. He would roll up the alarm in his blanket so people wouldn't hear it and he learned to switch off the button.

He had such bad dementia, but he could still figure out things like that! He figured out how to get out the front door. He thought his car was out there. He would ask Molly, "Where's my car?" He fell more than once so they finally devised another way to secure him. He fell again and had to be taken to the trauma center because he hit his head. Finally, they had him wear a helmet except when he was in bed. He was pretty good about wearing it. Though his dementia progressed a bit more rapidly he still had some good days. One day, the nurse at the facility called my daughter and said she wanted to send him to the emergency room because he had vomited some brown stuff that looked like coffee grounds. We allowed them to take him to the emergency room and it turned out he had a hernia in his stomach. It had been there for years and years and years but, for some strange reason, part of his intestines popped out and his hernia stopped the intestines from working. While the hernia was there, he didn't have surgery. They just popped it back in with their hands, but he got so upset and the dementia kicked in so strongly that they gave him medication to knock him out.

Molly was exploring every opportunity because she wanted to make sure she was doing everything possible for my husband. She didn't want him to suffer and decided to see about surgery to correct that hernia and the surgeon wouldn't do it because her father was 91. The surgeon didn't think he would make it through the surgery. I am 85 and my daughter is 53. When my husband woke up, the surgeon talked to him and tried to feed him. My husband took a bite and looked the surgeon straight in the face. He said, "No more," and refused to eat anymore. My husband died in 2016 at the age of 91. His death made the decision for my daughter.

I was becoming more and more forgetful and relying almost completely on Molly.

I went with her on a Study Abroad Program for her work and she took a caregiver with us because I couldn't stay by myself. We did that twice and then went to Hilton Head. On the way back, I asked my daughter, "Where is my mother?" Molly got scared but drove on. My daughter would keep me in her office where I had a special chair. I could even go to the bathroom by myself, but I thought my daughter was a bad person and ran out of the bathroom one day screaming at her.

[Molly says of herself. "To see both my mother, Trish. and my father diminish was terrible because they were such vibrant people. My mother's a people person, wrote, loved to talk, and now she just speaks gibberish. That was one of the first things I noticed. She loved to read and suddenly it was really hard and very scary. It was hard being a caregiver for both of them, yet extremely painful to put her in the facility, but she did not snap out of it. I paid out-of-pocket for a caretaker. I even had my mother sleep with me, but she became combative, telling me I was not her daughter. I felt really, really guilty about putting her in skilled nursing, but I had to work. Her downfall happened in 2017 and I'm not sure she knows who I am. Sometimes she will cry when she sees me but, oddly enough, I will ask, "Do you know who I am?" She will say, "No." I visit her every day unless I am in Italy and I pay out of pocket for a private aide four days a week for four hours because I want my mom to be very clean. I feel good that my mom is getting some individual attention. I'm not bashing the facility because there are some things that don't always work right. It could be so much worse. Anything that is done is not intentional. It's just that they don't have enough people working there. It is what it is. Residents aren't being ignored because the aides or nurses are nasty people. It's just too much and they can't do it all and that's my big complaint as it would be anywhere. It's clean here, it doesn't smell, and the staff is nice for the most part.]

Today, you can see me with a severe case of dementia, in a wheelchair. I have good days mostly when I can be around music and bad days when I seem to be searching, just roaming the halls, often without direction. I have a beautiful voice and especially love "How Great Thou Art" and can hit the high notes. Not many people can do that. Although my verbal skills are diminished, I can still say a few comprehensible words. My day is brighter when I see, and remember, my daughter Molly. She visits me every day, without fail.

"It is of the Lord's mercies that we are not consumed,
because His compassion's fail not."
– Lamentations 3:22

Patricia passed away Thanksgiving Day
November 26, 2020.

*Molly considered her "the most cherished and treasured mentor, best friend, and sacrificing
mother that a person could ever wish for."*

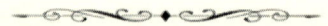

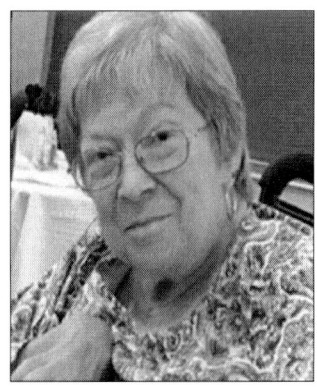

Irene Foster

Chapter 19 – The Bolins (Irene Foster)

A Quiet Force for God
Lynne and Pastor Barry Bolin's recollection of Irene Foster

"When my daughter and I met Irene, who had both legs amputated, we thought we would witness to her and lift her spirits. It was quite the opposite. Although severely disabled, Irene spoke to her faith and how she had not given up through her many trials. My daughter and I sat there with grateful tears after being in the presence of this quiet, soft-spoken, yet powerful woman of God."
– the Author

When Irene was around 15 years-old, she and I [Lynne] worked together downtown in Athens, Ohio, at a cafeteria. The owners were strange. One told you to do something and you had to do it. Then, the other one would turn around and tell you to do something different. So, we learned how to work really hard. We started in the kitchen. We began carrying trays and when you carried trays to the tables you had to take the tips and put them in a big tip jar for everybody. We worked in the kitchen together, learning how to cook, do the dishes, scrub the pots and pans, and clean everything that needed to be cleaned. After we learned all this stuff, we were allowed to work on the line. Sometimes we'd work a split shift and her dad would come and get us. I lived down on East State Street in Athens, not too far away, but he'd take us out to Shade, to his house. Irene and I used to go on catering jobs with the cafeteria owners and we had a ball together. Irene was so much fun to be around. I lost track of her after I got married and then when I saw her again, she was at a nursing home.

Barry (Lynne's husband) and I went to visit a friend who was dying and Irene was in the bed right next to our friend. I didn't recognize Irene. I knew she had Multiple Sclerosis (MS) because she was always asking people about Barry's nephew who had MS at the same time. She heard my voice and said, "Lynne?" I said, "Yes, who are you?" It was Irene. Barry would go visit her after that. I'd see her a few times, but then she moved to another facility. I was so glad to see her in there.

She had to get her legs amputated. She's prayed for me and I've prayed for her and every time we'd go on vacation, I'd bring her back a compact disc because she liked Gospel music. I always liked to bring something back to her because I knew she couldn't get out and go. I miss her. She was one of my favorites.

Born August 1, 1950, Irene was from Shade, Ohio. She loved her dad dearly. She and her dad were more compatible than Irene and her mother. Then I learned from Irene that when she got MS, her husband left her. He wouldn't stay. He wouldn't take care of her and it was hard for her to live at home and have her family take care of her, so she put herself into a nursing home.

Her faith? She knew Jesus a long time ago. She was a Christian when we worked together and I wasn't. She just believed and went to church all the time. Irene was a good person – a very, very, good person.

[Barry adds] She was in the nursing home for physical rehabilitation for a while. She was having some problems physically and would get urinary tract infections. When somebody's got MS, the infections were very toxic. She had arrived at the facility where I had started my devotions and preaching. This is something I'll never forget. The activities director, came to me and said, "Can you come back to see Irene? She wants to see you. We're calling the family and don't think she's got long to live." I closed my service quickly, grabbed her hand, and said, "Come with me." In the room, the director was on one side of the bed and I was on the other, and we both held her hands and Irene said, "Barry, I'm ready to see Jesus, I just need the transportation." I knew right away what she needed. I ran into that all the time – people being in the church for 50 years want that security, want to make sure of where they're going, and they want to have the right transportation. I went over the Romans Scripture with her. You know the one where all sinners come short of the glory of God, you ask Jesus to forgive your sins (Romans 3:23-24). I asked her, "Do you ask Jesus to forgive your sins?" She said, "Yes." I said, "Do you believe in your heart that Jesus Christ died on the cross for your sins and was resurrected?" "Yes, I do." I said, "Well that confirms your salvation, you're there." Those in the room looked at me as Irene's mouth went open. I said, "She's just at peace with the Lord because I see her breathing."

The next morning when I visited, Irene was sitting up in bed eating breakfast. We've always said she had nine lives. That was the first time and I ran into four or five other instances where she appeared to be close to death. The only thing different was she'd call me at home, I'd come in, and then she'd say, "I'm ready to see Jesus and I don't need the transportation." She became good friends with Margaret, who was one of the founders of Romans Road Church situated at the nursing home. Irene served with her on the Resident Council.

I think before she passed, she got a urinary tract infection again. She went up to Columbus and I went to see her. Her brothers were in the hallway and one said, "She's not going to make it back." I said, "Don't be surprised for she might." Long story short, she was back. I think they sent her back too soon from the hospital because she was still having problems when she returned. She contracted pneumonia, lost her voice, and finally she just started having bad sores on her legs. The sores were causing infections and she decided to have her legs amputated. She handled all of her sicknesses excellently.

Matter of fact, it was during April when we were going to Myrtle Beach as we always do. Her caretaker told me that Irene was going to have an amputation. She wanted us to go on to Myrtle Beach and said she would update us and keep in contact. I probably still have the text. We hadn't gotten back to West Virginia yet when I received a call saying it was a very serious operation – major. I asked how she was doing and was told I should ask her. Irene had just gotten out of recovery and she was on the phone. I said, "Irene, how are you doing?" She said, "Well, I lost about 10 pounds, but what a way to lose weight." [Lynne] That's how she took it. She was a marvelous person.

I think she relied on me [Barry] for a lot of information because I'd hear her tell other people, "I'm fine," or "Everything's fine." I'd look at her and say, "No, you're not. Tell me the truth. Don't lie to me." Then she'd tell me whatever problems she was having. That's the gist of most of the things with her.

[Lynne] She was just a happy-go-lucky person. She always cared about everybody else and she didn't want you to know what was happening to her.

[Barry] Her favorite Scripture was Isaiah 40:31. I was led to preach that one Sunday and that was the last time she heard it. That was the last service she attended. For some reason, I just felt like I needed to do that again. I actually did it over the radio and I thought, I'm just going to do that for Irene. She was a dandy for sure.

"But they that wait upon the Lord shall renew their strength; they shall mount up on wings as eagles; they shall run and not be weary, and they shall walk, and not faint."
– Isaiah 40:31

Irene was transported on January 26, 2019.

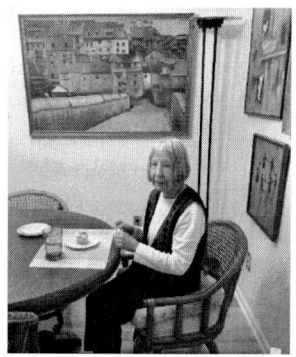

Marilyn Grier Davis

Chapter 20 – Stacia Davis Moore
(Marilyn Grier Davis)

Creative Entrepreneur
Stacia Davis Moore's recollections of her mother,
Marilyn Greer Davis

*"Coming back to Athens and seeing this site we built
and knowing the benefit and the premise of what that
community can mean to seniors' lives was promising.
At the same time, I was hearing a lot of long-time community folks beat it down and didn't want the facility.
I'm a believer in this facility and what this can mean,
and now I have seen it because I'm inside, too."*

I am Stacia, a 60 year-old divorcee who has traveled throughout the U.S. and a little in Canada. I am an only child and the only family member remaining since the death of my parents. My faith has been strong since I was quite young. I made a covenant to God to take care of my parents from a promise made very young, 10 years-old or so, and I'm very grateful. I think I made some sacrifices, but I'm here. I've learned a great, great deal and because of the two people who were my parents, I have had an exceptional walk on this earth.

I moved us to Athens in 2009 from Akron, Ohio. Back in 2002, we sold the family business and I modified part of the house, which was purchased because it was a studio. I turned that into my parents' living space because I wasn't able to keep the studio business. So, that just confirmed the commitment that I had made at such a young age. Maybe because having two grandparents on both sides was very important. They were present in my life. My dad's parents and my folks purchased land side by side to build. They decided not to build and that spot moved just a little bit. Then they bought another closure of land and each built their own homes. They were unique homes as they were built – artistic and creative –and when my dad's parents died, I was very present, and my mother's parents came and bought that property and lived in it.

Then, Florida beckoned and I went there a lot because my grandparents were going quite often. I would stay in Florida in retirement communities and got to know people from all over the country. So, I've watched the healthcare system up close. I also had an aunt, a great aunt, who was in the Chapel Hill area and she ended up in one of the earlier retirement communities, the earliest in North Carolina. I was watching and learning about that concept before it really hit Ohio. Coming back to Athens and seeing this site we built and knowing the benefit and the premise of what that community can mean to seniors' lives was promising. At the same time, I was hearing a lot of long-time community folks beat it down and didn't want the facility. I'm a believer in this facility and what this can mean and now I have seen it because I'm inside, too.

I was taking a walk around the neighborhood where we lived. My parents were out; they were often away. I was on my own from a very young age. They were very active and there were some seniors who cared for me at the time, but I was often alone. I was walking that path and I asked, "Why am I here? I'm not needed, I'm not really an active kid." You know, I'm more of an adult than I am a kid. I've always been around adults, not kids. They had moved, when I was 10 years-old, from one community into another and that was stark, a hard transition, and I just felt the presence say, "Care for them and I will provide for you."

My grandfather had oral cancer when I was about five years-old. At that time, treatment was pretty radical in the Columbus hospital. I would often walk over to the hospital to the long-term care space and spend time with him. I was very young. My grandmother would sit on the couch in the library at home crocheting, drinking bourbon and beer, and watching the Cleveland Indians. That was her pattern and we were close. She was creative and influential. My parents again were out and I got a phone call from my grandmother that she had fallen. I immediately ran over and found her on the floor. She had stood up, her hip let go, and I called the ambulance to get her into care. I always seemed to have been present in that way. I was present for my grandfather, too – more of a distant spirit. He was passing and he made a point to phone me. He was still quite cognizant when he said, "I know it's coming." I whispered, "You know it's okay." He said, "But I wanted you to make it down again." I said, "Well, I'm not able to, but you're okay and I'm okay, so go." He did. It was always just that knowing, I guess.

Both parents showed signs of dementia before moving to Athens. Dad seemed to be a little more focused, but I could see it with mom, too, because she was having struggles with the checkbook and keeping up with things she had always done before. During the process of moving from Akron to Athens, I had moved my folks into a duplex and I was making another run to Akron with mom. Dad had a stroke that was slight and not particularly significant in a visual way, but it changed him and changed his personality which often comes with dementia in the last years. His was disoriented more because of cardiovascular issues and Chronic Obstructive Pulmonary Disease (COPD). Mom, born April 13, 1931, followed more in the way of Alzheimer's, but her parents had passed when she was quite young, and so there was no history to know.

Dad got up one morning at three o'clock and decided it was time to make coffee, get dressed, and go to work. I got a frantic call that he had fallen putting on his pants. He broke his hip and perforated his bowel. Within a week-and-a-half, we had gone through the first surgery, local anesthetic, but the bowel issue wasn't identified. At the point when surgery was discussed, it did not seem practical with what his wish would be and had always been discussed. Death was always talked about openly. End of life planning was a part of their action and, in fact, they led that in the community and got lawyers looking at the topic long before it was common. He passed in 2014 and I moved over into their side of the duplex about a year later.

I was accepting work at a nursing home and caring for mom through her life's end. She broke her hip nine months before she passed. The disease was certainly a present factor for her experience and, in the end, a seizure was the last couple of steps in her final week of passing away. Watching that progress of going from the person that you know is in there to seeing her diminish in memory and in health was an opportunity to try and learn, to focus, and to be educated. I've read extensively. I've discussed extensively. I prayed. What could I possibly do with what time I would have left, knowing the likelihood of an experience with dementia was growing as I was watching this in both of them? I came up with two words of "what" and "where" was my passion?

One passion was creativity and the other one was aging. I came up with my mission statement of, "To share and learn all I know and learn about creativity and aging." It's been an insightful experience. My dad and mom knew I was studying and they were grateful, I think, to be at home. They were grateful to see all of the effort I applied to keeping them at home. It's not an easy process and, if I had been working, it would have been impossible, even with a spouse. It was their walk and so as long as I could continue to come to them with positive energy, whether they knew in the end who I was or not, really did not matter. I knew. As long as they were happy, they were in a better space for transition than not being happy.

As far as a support system for me as an only child, I don't know specifically and I don't seek specifically. My hope is to stay as tactfully engaged as I can in two ways: One is creating work that comes from my heart because that is a big part of what keeps my energy high and keeps me well; and two is being able to continue to be very engaged in my own work, creative expression, and helping others until I realize that I'm not capable to do that.

We come to wonder for a while but eventually we come to realize. Whether we accept dementia or not is the question, but I think I would be the exception and, at that point, I guess I'm thinking more like Native Americans in the long walk. I don't care to leave a burden. I hope to deplete as much of the material things I've collected and turn them into something with creation and expression so that there's not much left. That's where I feel I need to be responsible. For me, at this time, I need enough cash flow and income to prevent me from being a burden in our society the ways things are structured.

I think as I walk the compounds where I live now, I'm in joy to be in that space with lots of memories that are good. But, it's also an opportunity to create some new moments. There's so much that I don't need. There's so much there, right? Yet I'm not compelled yet to let go. There are too many glasses, there are too many plates, too many pots, etc. The space is allowing, so I'm not compelled to let it all go. Some of the items are beautiful items that mom collected. I love keeping them around, but it's a mess.

My mother was exceptionally fortunate to have extended family to immediately care for her when her mother died tragically in a fire. Friends of that extended family, who were childless, asked to adopt her and did. Those folks became grandparents to me which enabled my mother to pursue a degree in education at Ohio State University and allowed for the meeting between my dad and my mom.

Mom taught for seven or eight years in elementary – third, and fourth grades. She did a tremendous amount of volunteer work and a great deal of card playing, earning national points and leading a lot of that activity in the community. She developed really great friendships, creating a social structure for her and my dad in weekend couples' activity. And those brain muscles are the strongest muscles, I've heard, so she continued to play cards long into the experience of dementia. There was joy in that for dad as well and we simplified the game but that was still an important part of it. She was independent and she drove independence in me. They put me on a bus and on a train when I was about five years-old to go to Columbus to visit family and there was a lot of travel because of the business. We were fortunate to get to go places. Our business was a company that designed, engineered, and manufactured load-lifting equipment. After 9/11, things started to change and we were really on that ride of change.

My mom and dad probably said more about me than I ever heard. They weren't very open and complimentary but were certainly respectful. They seemed to, as I look back, treat me as an adult individual at a very early age and stepped back from a role of parenting. Now, nobody knows how to parent when they become parents. So, lately, I'm just so grateful for how they did handle me. My dad loved music. Big band music was a part of our home and we made sure to accomplish putting on a lot of shows. I listen to music now. My dad wanted to be an architect and start a business. There was creativity on both of their sides which really helped and developed me, too. They had a lot of beautiful things and they explored and shared much of their life with me. I have a really great warm glow when I think of each of them together and I think I had a charmed life in that they seemed to be solid as a couple and so few are having that experience today. I did not have that experience.

If my mother could change anything about her life, I think that she might have really wanted to know her parents more. I feel there was always a sense of loss there and a lack of connection. I often reminded her how very fortunate she was for the family who did come into her life. Yes, there were hardships and, no, we weren't in a society at a point where we analyzed, studied, healed, you know, and brought people through pain. That said, though, there were suffering and hardships, but what a wonderful outcome in how God supported her. The parallel in my life, between them being at home and my working and seeing the day-to-day health care, I'd rather stay home with my parents.

The first glaring thing in nursing homes is a lack of prepared servers. We are understaffed in all regards and, in a moment of crisis, we are going to be short. I've done my part to try and raise that awareness and no amount of warning is really helping us to prepare for this situation. I think that we need all aspects fully staffed, not just here but every nursing home. We need home health care, we need assisted living to be available, but I also know that we need long-term care. All should be high-quality. There's no excuse for anything less and is there more that can be done? Absolutely. It's a major, major movement in this moment in time and we can't neglect, we can't not make noise, and we must insist on that quality. We do a pretty good job here.

One of the things that would make a difference is to build more unity amongst staff and allow for a higher level of understanding and respect amongst all staff. If we have that net of compatibility and companionship, we would then be better servers for our residents. Lacking that or anything less than being supportive and open is only going to create detriment across the board. The souls who are here and coming here to help as servers, need more, and it isn't simply economics. They definitely need more economics, but they need a little more because they're giving heart and soul and body, and burning out from what they're doing and they become a part of the need. We're often missing the point in all of what's happening here in a humanistic sense.

Now if you took it over to an economic sense, I think we're missing the point there, too. For every entry, for every loss, for every turnover, the costs are instrumentally high and I don't think we're looking at those. If we were, I think we would see a shift and improvement, but I think that shift has to come in conjunction with the level of openness, the level of compassion and caring, support, and comradery. We need to have those qualities rather than feeling threatened or a lack of trust, or overspent, and we need downtime. People who are doing this work need to be whole. This journey has been a pop-up part of my passion and I don't know what comes next because I'm on this thing right here.

God and only God is why I have a mission statement and whether I'm active or not. The time out that I took to focus solely on my mother and my father was simply gaining and gathering more understanding and depth. Where I will be positioned is beyond my knowing at this time, but four or five years ago it took me out of the State of Ohio, to the Ohio Arts Council, to the Department of Aging. It allowed me to go to Columbus to meetings on aging through the American Association of Retired Persons (AARP), and to go to Washington, D.C. to work on one little aspect which is creative aging. I lost the freedom and capability to continue on that project. I hope I'm able to do more.

"Whatever your hand finds to do, do it with thy might."
– Ecclesiastes 9:10

Stacia's mother passed February 18, 2019.

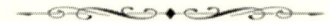

Chapter 21 – Man of Action

Interviewee prefers to remain anonymous
Written by the author

In social animals, the highest ranking individual is sometimes designated as the Alpha. An Alpha male is a man who takes charge no matter what the situation.

This gentleman is wise, all knowing, commands attention, takes up space, the first to volunteer and, upon occasion, bossy. Yet, he can be most sociable, helpful, and amenable.

When the war came in the '40s, and his family was in an internment camp, all he remembers about the camp is that he was deeply afraid of dogs. After the war, he moved to Fayetteville, Ohio, then to Cincinnati. After graduating from the University of Cincinnati's College of Engineering as a chemical engineer, he worked as an application research chemist, food chemist, and land developer in Ohio and Pennsylvania.

Both parents were born in San Jose, California. Each of their five children was born in a different city – Santa Barbara, Long Beach, or Los Angeles in California; Mariemont, or Cincinnati in Ohio. The interviewee married a Cincinnatian, and they have two sons and two daughters who live in different states.

He worked as an application research scientist, testing products to see how they could be used. Also, as a creator of cellulose inventions, he used ground-up newspapers to make fireproof products and developed uses for front-end loaders. Sugar, salt, and pepper packaging were among his designs along with a 200-gallon container to make jelly.

He chose his current care facility because, as a volunteer with a singing group, he loved the environment and the care that the residents were given. As his health declined in 2017, it became evident that everyday care was necessary. It was best to become a permanent resident because a condition affecting his motion was causing frequent falls.

He doesn't believe he's lost a great deal other than motion. He still enjoys the support of his wife whom he married in 1962. She lives nearby and their children and five grandchildren are very much in his life. He loves his wife, food, singing, and card games. What matters most to him at the facility are meeting people and becoming friends. His hobbies include photography and gardening.

"For I know the plans for you," declares the Lord, "plans to prosper you and not to harm you, plans to give you a hope and a future."
—Jeremiah 29:11

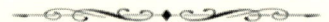

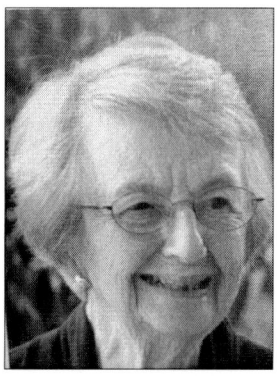

Lelia Bess Brownlee Relyea

Chapter 22 – Dorothy Relyea Schey (Bess Relyea)

Family First
Written by the author after interviewing Dorothy Relyea
Schey about her mother, Bess Relyea

"She believes in the value in the family and loves joyful music."

Bess was born June 27, 1925, in Calhoun, Georgia, and majored in nutrition at the University of Georgia. She is 93 years-old and widowed. Her husband passed away in October 2012. Bess enjoyed traveling and she's been to a number of state capitols, and to England and Spain. She had been at The Maplewood before coming to her current facility.

Bess has three children, two boys and one girl, and loves her family and friends. Dorothy says, "She believes in the value in the family and loves joyful music. She loves the facility she is in because of the very nice people and how they take very good care of her. Some days are better than others. She's had to use the sit-to-stand equipment to get up but can't do any walking. She seems to be happy and especially likes aide Virginia. She has her kinfolk coming regularly and her health care assistant, Linda, is a good friend and looks after her.

"My brother Doug," says Dorothy, "lives closer than either I or my other brother does and he sees mom weekly, sometimes daily. Before COVID, he was a fixture at the facility not only helping her but helping others as well.

"My mother has been here since 2013 and is blessed to have lots of good friends. She's lost a lot of people, though, and laments over that from time to time. She loves good conversation, music, and has a sense of humor. My dad, her husband, was an independent insurance agent and he won lots of trips that enabled them to travel – wonderful travel. She absolutely loves Coca Cola, too.

"What is so difficult for me and my brothers with her aging and losing strength is we never thought she'd become the 'child' where we would have to take care of her and make the decisions. Mom has faith in God and I know there is no place that is perfect. I'm the advocate now and I had no idea this is how life would be as you get older."

And He walks with me, and He talks with me,
and He tells me I am His own –
from In the Garden (1912) by C. Austin Miles.

Bess passed away July 23, 2019.

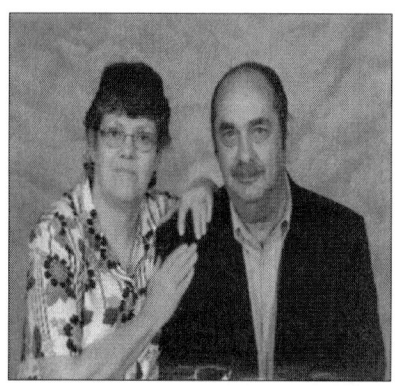

Lynne and Barry Bolin

Chapter 23 – Pastor Barry Bolin, Lynne Bolin, and Bill and Barbara Bolin Miller

Written by the author after interviewing Pastor Barry and Lynne Bolin, Romans Road Church

"Every nursing and rehab center should have the Bolins, selflessly giving of themselves and of their substance."
– the Author

Pastor Barry Bolin is married to Lynne Berry Bolin and is from Albany, Ohio. He's 73 years-old, retired from pastoring at established, denominational churches, and is dedicated to pastoral ministry in nursing homes and hospitals. Both of his parents are deceased, as are his two brothers and one sister. One sister, Barbara, lives in a nursing facility. He said what makes this one different from other facilities are the care and cleanliness.

His professional vocation was regional director for the American Federation of State, County & Municipal Employees (AFSCME) from which he retired in 2006. He is a high school graduate and was president of the class of 1964. He went to work immediately after high school and visited every state in the United States after retirement.

Prior to graduation from high school, so many of his classmates were focusing on attending business college in Columbus, Ohio. He was offered a job at a market in Athens as frozen foods manager so, instead of going to business school, he accepted the job as manager with good pay and benefits. After several years there, he was hired at a mental health center and, after working there for 10 years, retired as a psychiatric aide supervisor and next was hired by AFSCME. He retired from AFSCME after 22 years.

Retirement helped him return to various travels and ministries. He felt led to get back into more church work with a van ministry, on the finance committee, and with other committees. Barry served as a faith builder leader and adult senior Sunday School teacher for seven years. His desire for deeper studies led him to take university studies and he became an ordained licensed non-denominational minister. A hands-on blessing was completed in Greenville, South Carolina. Pastor Bolin developed a planet church in Athens as the Romans Road with help from several residents at a facility.

*"That if thou shalt confess with thy mouth the Lord Jesus,
and believe in thy heart that God hath
raised him from the dead, thou salt be saved."
– Romans 10:9*

*Lynne Bolin
Weekly Bible Study Teacher*

"Power grabs can be draining."

Lynne is a 69-year-old Athens native who worked as a housekeeper and is now semi-retired. She graduated from high school and worked cleaning restaurants, the hospital, and the welfare department in Athens. She's been to Canada, Puerto Rico, Mexico, Prince Edward Island the Virgin Islands, and all over the United States.

Lynne has one child from a previous marriage and never thought of herself as one in ministry. She was always the helper or the "help meet" person in the background and did a lot by feeding people and providing clothes. She told a story about a particular church in which she was involved where the clothing program was going so well that the pastor actually got jealous and took control of everything. "Power grabs can be draining," says Lynne. She finally quit that ministry after being there for a while. "The entire clothing program went downhill because of one man's need to be given credit for something he did not do."

She never thought she would be teaching Bible study because she didn't see herself in the role of teaching or ministry, but always in the background. "But God called me to start teaching each week at the facility and as I began the studies, the attendance began to grow. I then joined hand-in-hand with my husband in nursing home ministry."

"Thy Word is a lamp unto my feet and a light unto thy path." –
Psalm 119:105

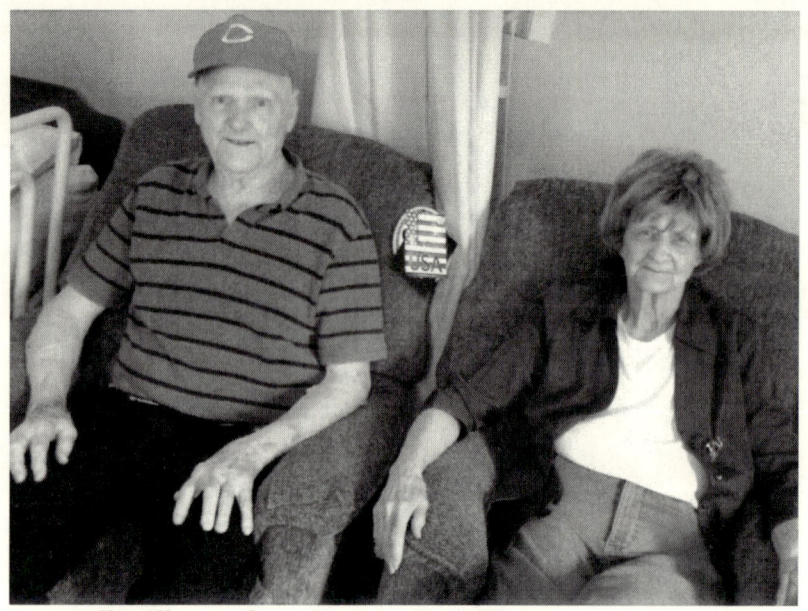

Bill Miller and Barbara Bolin Miller (Barry's Sister)
Nursing Home Residents
Love at First Sight as told to the author
Married 68 Years

"I saw her in a parking lot in Athens and she was so beautiful
that I just wanted to hug her. I told her she had a flat tire. She
didn't. I just didn't want her to leave because I wanted to see her.
She looked at it and when she stood up, I hugged her.
We were married one week later." – Bill Miller

The story of Barbara and Bill Miller cannot be told separately for they have been together for 68 years and are even in the same room at a nursing home facility – the only couple. Barbara was born January 6, 1934, and is Pastor Barry Bolin's sister. She was a 1952 graduate of Albany High School. Her past employment includes a grocery store in Albany, Sears in Athens, and the Vinton County Court House where she helped abused children. She attended Albany Baptist Church for many years and, while at the nursing home, attended and was a member of Romans Road Church. She was an accomplished pianist and singer.

She and Bill had two children; both have passed. Bill worked in a grocery store, and for an insurance company. He is a high school graduate with one year of college. Barbara and Bill lived in Bisbee, Arizona, for many years. They went there because of their daughter's asthma. While in Bisbee, Bill worked in the copper mines and also was in the Navy four years as a store clerk.

William E. Miller continues to reside in a facility and misses Barbara deeply since she passed away. They were the model couple – never one without the other.

"... in sickness and in health, to love and to cherish, forsaking all others, for as long as you both shall live."

Barbara passed away November 17, 2020.

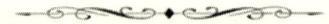

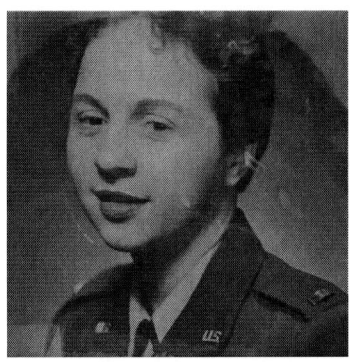

Betty Higgins

Chapter 24 – Betty Higgins

Air Force Veteran and Retired Nurse tells her story

"The hardest part is the loneliness."

I grew up in a little town called Natrona, Pennsylvania, where I was born, and we just lived in an old wooden house because that's all anybody could afford. I have a book from Natrona. I went to nursing school there, and I have pictures from nursing school, too. My roommate sent me a book and it shows me and her at the May Day celebration. We were part of the court as attendants. There were quite a few of us including our queen Virginia. I don't know where she is now. Most of them are dead and gone.

We had coal mining and the steel mill there. Now, I can't remember what the census was, but we had three or four schools, playgrounds, churches and, of course, a hospital and a fire department. Because when you are little, you don't get too excited about anything. Back then, the generations were different than they are now. We always tried to make friends with certain girls or boys from the Catholic school so that we had somebody to call for help or if we wanted to go somewhere or to get to school. I left there and went to the public school which was hard work because it was larger and it offered more subjects than the Catholic school did.

I wanted to fly and joined the Air Force and went to college for nursing. I figured I would do nursing school and then go to college. We didn't have a television, but something inspired me to want to pin on the white hat and wear the starched white uniform to help others. I was a registered nurse when I went into the service. I went into the service because I wanted to fly but then I chickened out on that. I didn't think I would have the ability to jump out of a plane into the ocean. It was too scary. I originally wanted to fly commercially, but the commercial airlines said I was too fat. The service took me right in. There was no hesitation at all. When you're so young, your parents had to sign for you. My dad said, "I'm right here," and it was just that quick.

I lived in Glouster, Ohio, while I was still married. The worst day was when the children went off to college. I couldn't handle the big house and one day I fell and broke my hip. After that fall, while I was recuperating, neither my daughter nor my son had room for me, so I had to decide if I wanted to try to rent a place or go to a nursing home. I didn't take much time to decide. I wish I had. I wish I had taken time to figure out what I was going to do, but I just didn't. I ended up here.

The newer, local facility is one of the better places in this area for a nursing home but they're all so expensive and so lonely without family. You can check out apartments and see what they would cost, but you won't have anybody to really take care of you. If I fall here or if I get sick, they automatically call my children and let them know. So, the best part about being here is just that you've got someone to take care of you. I don't have to worry about paying the bills, the taxes, and that sort of thing. I like being outside in the beautiful courtyard. The hardest part is the loneliness. Yeah, the loneliness with no kids to talk with every day.

I worked at the state hospital in Athens. When I was working there it was just called The Asylum. That's another good piece of landscape owned by the university. We used to have everything there. They had cows, chickens, and planted all kinds of vegetables. They planted poinsettias and the one man who planted them would get them ready for Christmas, and then he would sell them and plant something else for the next season. That place was self-sufficient, but they had let it go because they weren't making enough money. They sold it and the state hospital moved to somewhere along the river.

I simply applied for the state hospital job. I wanted the three-to-11 shift because I wanted to be with my kids as much as I could. I was out of the service and worked at the hospital in Athens, but the head honcho didn't like me and got rid of me. I worked in Nelsonville for a while and they wanted to put me in positions for which I had no training. I said, "No, that's ridiculous." So, they said, "Well, we can't use you." I decided to go somewhere else where they will use me with the registered nurses' training I had.

At the hospital, I said to my boss, "I just can't get up that early. Could you use me on three-to-11 shift?" She said, "Oh, yes. That's the hardest shift." I took it and worked those hours the whole time I was there. I liked it and I learned a whole lot about myself and other people with whom I worked. But I couldn't handle that early day shift and the night shift. I couldn't stay awake on the night shift and on the day shift I couldn't get up early enough to make it on time. With three-to-11, I could sleep in as late as I wanted, watch the programs I wanted to watch, and go to work. It was really nice for me and my boss was a real good Director of Nursing.

Side Bar: Becoming a nurse is one of the most selfless acts a person can undertake. In a society of so many different races, cultures, customs, and beliefs, nurses are a universal gift to all, and the dedicated work that they do and kindness they deliver on a daily basis should serve as a reminder of the fundamental humanity inside us all. – Author Unknown

I liked what they did at The Asylum with the farm. The animals provided food and so on and so forth. And then they have places like this. My mother ended up in a nursing home because she got diabetes and couldn't take care of herself at all. She didn't want to live with me or my sister. She wanted to live with her oldest boy. She ended up being in the hospital and eventually both legs were cut off because of diabetes. She was in a nursing home for nine years. I went to see her whenever I could but to drive by myself from here to Pennsylvania was hard. I did it but if I had been smart enough, I could have taken the kids with me because my daughter is a good map reader. I wasn't afraid of the driving; it was just a long trip to take by myself – a good six hours.

When I turned 80, my daughter and grandchild made up a big box. There were 80 presents wrapped individually – one for each year. Some were little and some were big, so I said, "What did you do all of that for?" "Because we wanted to," she said. Even now she sends me stuff on my birthday. She is just very thoughtful that way.

After my husband left and I was trying to get over him, I met another gentleman and we went together for a long time. When he died, I was really betwixt and between and I never felt good about anything after that. He reminded me so much of my dad. He was very attentive and we did a lot together. I met him at the VFW on a bet. We both were military and I was working at the state hospital. Some nurses bet me that I wouldn't go have a drink with the guys and I went. I never drank alcohol and the drink I had was orange juice. He was excited that I didn't drink because he said that was what messed up his marriage – the alcohol. He was lonesome and I was lonesome. His wife was dead and my husband was married to someone else. My kids encouraged me. If I could do it all over, I would do things differently, but you can't go back.

I went to get my COVID vaccine in that beautiful new medical building on the university's campus. They took us in the van. I don't know what was there before in that space because I haven't been to Athens for a while. Once they take your car away from you, that is that. My kids are out-of-state so they are not around to take me anywhere, but the only place I'd want to go would be a place to eat or go to a good movie. Things have changed so. When this virus popped up it's different. It's just one of those things, I guess.

I cannot go any place now without help and the fact that I can't get out and drive anymore is like you're just out in the desert somewhere and isolated. And especially with this COVID now. I am always going to have the football games, "Go Steelers!," she cheers, and basketball on television and it's really hard to cut everything off.

If I could change anything in my life, I would change my health. I would want no broken bones and I would want to drive to see the kids. I have one great grandchild and she's cute as can be. My memory is not what it used to be at all and it's so embarrassing. They live out of state and they're getting older like me.

My advice when one has to come to a nursing home is to check out nursing homes closer to their family. They're all similar and they all have problems with staff. They have to do things that most people wouldn't think about doing for people.

"Wait on the Lord: be of good courage, and he shall strengthen thine heart: wait, I say, on the Lord."
– Psalm 27:14

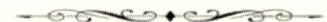

Chapter 25 – Nursing Home Staffing

Nursing home reports to the federal government indicate staffing was less than reported, according to federal data and adding to what many families experience as lacking in what is necessary to meet the needs of residents (Nursing Home Reform Modernization Act of 2020 (currently in Congressional Committee).

Records reveal frequent fluctuations in daily staffing with the weekends being particularly sparse. At average facilities, personnel cared for nearly twice as many residents as they did when there were more staff. Statistics analyzed by Kaiser Health News (2018), come from daily payroll records. Medicare just recently began gathering and publishing data from more than 14,000 nursing homes, as required by the Affordable Care Act of 2010.

Kaiser found payroll records offer strong evidence that the federal government's five-star rating system for nursing homes often exaggerated staffing levels and rarely identified times when staffing was lean. Medicare relies on the new data to evaluate staffing, but the revamped star ratings still mask the fluctuating levels of people working on a day to day basis. At several of the facilities in which the author has received care, one can roam the halls looking for an aide who might already be overloaded with work. The call light goes on and it could be several minutes to 30 minutes, or more, when someone shows up at the door. It's rare when someone responds to a light right away.

With the nationwide crisis of staff shortages, aides hustle to deliver meals, feed those who cannot feed themselves, get residents to the bathroom, change soiled linens and residents' clothing, pick up trays, and respond to those who habitually put their call lights on because they are lonely or just need to talk. It is evident workers are overburdened and underpaid for the essential life-saving tasks they do such as helping to avoid bed sores by regularly changing the position of a patient to avert issues in a timely manner that could lead to infection or hospitalization.

The gaps in care change. Some weekday duties are regular such as dressing, bathing, and eating. Routines might change on the weekends when there are not as many activities. Administrators often argue not as many workers are needed on the weekends because of the change in schedules – less in-house activities and more family members visiting. Medicare does not set a minimum resident-to-staff ratio, but it does require the presence of a registered nurse for eight hours a day and a licensed nurse at all times.

According to Kaiser, facilities that Medicare rated positively for staffing levels on its Nursing Home Compare Web site, were short nurses and aides on some days. On its best-staffed days, one facility had one aide for every eight residents, while on its lowest-staffed days the ratio was one-to-18. Nursing levels also varied.

The Centers for Medicare & Medicaid Services oversee nursing home inspections and said in a statement that it "is concerned and taking steps to address fluctuations in staffing levels" that have emerged from the new data. Medicare & Medicaid said it would lower ratings for nursing homes that had gone seven or more days without a registered nurse. Payroll records examined by Kaiser showed staffing levels similar to those it had reported before. A chief operating officer of a for-profit chain said in a statement that his facility has enough nurses and aides to properly care for its 120 residents. "But this facility," he noted, "like other nursing homes, is in 'a constant battle' to recruit and retain employees even as it has increased pay to be more competitive. Weekend staffing is a special challenge as employees are guaranteed every other weekend off." Paydays and vacations also leave facilities operating at bare bone levels.

Daily payroll reports to calculate average staffing ratings, begun by the federal government in 2018, replaced the old method of relying on nursing homes to report staffing for the two weeks before an inspection. Kaiser says, "The homes sometimes anticipated when an inspection would happen and could staff up before it. The new records show that on at least one day during the last three months of 2017 – the most recent period for which data were available – a quarter of facilities reported no registered nurses at work."

Studies have found nursing homes with lower staffing tended to have more health code violations – another crucial measure of quality, according to the Kaiser report. "Even with more reliable data, Medicare's five-star rating system still has shortcomings. Medicare still assigns stars by comparing a home to other facilities, essentially grading on a curve. As a result, many homes have kept their rating even though their payroll records showed lower staffing than before. Also, more than 1,000 facilities remain unrated by Medicare, either because of data anomalies or because they were too new to have a staffing history."

What are optimal staffing levels? There is no consensus. Medicare will not respond to requests asking for those level saying in 2016 that it preferred that facilities "make thoughtful, informed staffing plans" based on the needs of residents. However, since 2014, Kaiser finds health inspectors have cited one in eight nursing homes for having too few nurses and states, "With nurse assistants earning an average of $13.23 an hour in 2017, nursing homes compete for workers not only with better-paying employers like hospitals, but also with retailers. Understaffing leads predictably to higher turnover."

This author sees it every day. Aides don't like the long hours when they have to work over to the next shift due to call offs, shortages, and administrative inflexibility for dealing with family issues, a death, or a school schedule. I agree with a man in the Kaiser study whose mother lived at a nursing facility until her death and said, "They get burned out and they quit. It's been constant turmoil, and it never ends." The Kaiser study observed Medicare's payroll records for the nursing homes which showed that there were, on average, 11% fewer nurses providing direct care on weekends and 8% fewer aides. Staffing levels fluctuated substantially during the week as well, the report added, when an aide at a typical home might have to care for as few as nine residents or as many as 14.

A retired teacher whose elderly wife lives in a facility says staffing levels have long seemed inadequate. He and a group of other residents and family members became so dissatisfied that they formed a council to scrutinize the home's operation. Medicare requires nursing home administrators to listen to such councils' grievances and recommendations. "Almost every problem we've had on the floor is one that could have been alleviated with enough well-trained staff," said one family member. The facility declined to discuss individual residents but said it had investigated complaints and did not find inadequate staffing on those days. "Weekends are terrible," the family member said. While he's regularly there overseeing his wife's care, he wondered about the other residents who don't have people to visit or advocate.

Chapter 26 – The COVID-19 Pandemic

And then the virus hit...

Who knew something like this would hit in our lifetime? There have been epidemics before and nationwide scares but, in this century of technological advances and discoveries, no one expected a virus that would, as of this writing, kill over 700,000 people of all demographics and cultures in the United States alone.

The keys to survival were, and still is, sanitizing, hand washing, social distancing, wearing masks and, later, testing, and vaccines. A model case was the facility in which I was doing rehabilitation. Right at the beginning of the spread in the United States, the administration placed the facility on lockdown. I wrote about it and the column was published in the local newspaper May 21, 2020.

COVID-19: An Insider's Look at Skilled Care

Forefront in the news are the deaths of our elderly population in skilled nursing homes during the COVID-19 pandemic. Ninety percent of residents have a recorded disability. One-third of U.S. COVID-19 deaths are in nursing homes. The nursing home industry was in trouble before COVID-19 struck. For years, nursing homes have struggled to attract new residents, faced high staffing turnover rates and shortages, and often operated on thin margins with little room to upgrade their facilities. How, then, does one who is a partaker of medical services in a skilled nursing home and rehabilitation facility feel, particularly now? Cautious. Distrustful. Afraid of infection. Isolated. The worst part is prolonged separation from family and friends. Add to this a disability and the issues are compounded. A person with any kind of disabling condition, unless fairly independent, needs close-up care on a daily basis – at home or in a facility. I've been on both sides of the coin. In 1995, I was paralyzed as the result of a benign spinal cord tumor. Following surgery to remove it (11 hours) and months of intense physical, occupational, recreational, and pool rehabilitation, I regained my mobility. Over the years, however, my strength decreased, and I would need more care and rehabilitation for short periods of time that increasingly became longer. Since 1995, I have been in at least seven hospitals and six skilled nursing/rehabilitation facilities. I've experienced the best and the worst. I write today, in the midst of nursing home tragedies everywhere to commend The Laurels in Athens (Ohio) for working diligently to keep residents in long-term care safe as well as those who come for rehabilitation. When the first positive case hit the facility in December 2020, it wasn't because the staff didn't do all they could to avoid it. Two weeks before the Governor (Ohio) announced the State's shut down, the facility began austere measures. Every employee coming and going uses only one door in the building to enter and exit which is monitored, has their temperature taken and recorded, signs in and out, and affirms no sickness present. All staff, no exceptions, change street clothes into laundered uniforms, swipe their shoes on a disinfectant mat, and wear an N-95 mask from the time they leave their vehicle to the time they return after a shift. The facility is known for its cleanliness and extra measures are taken with all surfaces. Packages are disinfected and placed in a dedicated room for 14 days before passing on and incoming letters are cleaned carefully. Gatherings for activities are suspended (even Bingo!) except for in-room activities or clusters of three or four with appropriate distancing. Therapy follows the same principles – only two or three residents in the gym at the same time with distancing. Residents must wear masks when out of their rooms and employees cannot bring items from home. Food is provided at the facility. Needless to say, hand washing is the utmost. Sound like prison? Perhaps. I see it as preventative. These actions not only protect the staff and the residents, but also the families of the staff they return home to each day. Most difficult is not being able to see loved ones and friends except through your windowpane. There is hope though. A skilled nursing and rehabilitation center in Belpre, Ohio, recently created a "visitation station" allowing families to somewhat reunite with their loved ones through Plexiglass panels that create a safe environment. To further protect its residents, the facility (The Laurels) dedicated one unit for those returning from brief hospital stays. They are separated for 14 days before going to another dedicated hall. Yes, there are issues with just about every facility on any given day minus the pandemic. Yet others could benefit by taking a few pages out of the Administrator's, the Director of Nursing's, and the team's playbook. A debt of gratitude is owed to the dedicated staff in all departments – housekeeping, laundry, maintenance, kitchen, rehabilitation, activities, nursing, nurses' aides, social services, administration – who work tirelessly to provide caring, quality service, and to keep us safe.

Well, when the virus hit the nursing home in December 2020 and sections of the facility were cordoned off for those who tested positive, it was a sad day. The stay in the first isolation unit was 14 days and then another 14 days in the second one. Staff and residents were tested twice each week and the vaccines began in January 2021. The isolation staff from housekeepers to nurses wore the full white "moon suit" gear.

I was ever so careful beyond the protocols. I asked one of my aides, "How will I know if I have COVID?" "When the white suits come for you," he said. I did have the sniffles for about a week, had my test one day, my vaccine the next, and two days later I had no sense of smell. I had COVID! How? I barely left my room, yet, there I was – isolated for two weeks. Those of us at the facility with the virus were blessed to get the

Remdesivir infusion and the appropriate medications. Residents at hundreds of other nursing facilities were not as blessed. My sense of smell returned after five days and all was well in preparation for getting my second vaccination. I'm thankful I had no lasting effects from COVID.

.

Chapter 27 – COVID-19 Exposed Staff Shortages in Nursing Homes

But the problem isn't new.

A report from CNN tells of experiences inside a specific nursing home where, as the COVID virus spread to its residents, people were regularly transported out to hospitals because of low oxygen supplies and as staff became infected, exacerbating already-low staffing levels. Staff concerned about their own health resigned and left the facility; others died.

A professor emerita at a California university said, "It's not surprising that they weren't able to cope with it." Recruiting and retaining staff wasn't easy before COVID because the hours are long, the workload is heavy, and the wages are low. An aide once told this author, "I don't have to put up with this. Although nursing care is good for my career path, I can go to a fast food restaurant, make more money, and have time for myself and my family." The average annual wage for nursing assistants – most of whom work full-time – in nursing care facilities is $30,120, according to the U.S. Bureau of Labor Statistics.

Says the CNN report, a certified nursing assistant lamented, "It was so few of us in the building that we were just literally running from floor to floor seeing who needed help. It was an absolute nightmare." More than 132,000 residents and more than 1,900 staff members died nationwide as of June 13, 2021, according to the Centers for Medicare & Medicaid Services (CMS). It is still unclear whether some deaths were actually from COVID or from loneliness, lack of regular activities, isolation, lack of contact with friends and family members, or fear of what was occurring,

As an insider who was blessed to have regular contact with family and friends through Facetime or Zoom, or writing, reading, and teaching to keep me occupied, I saw the quick demise of residents who experienced the wrath of the virus whether physically or mentally.

A June 2021 survey from the American Health Care Association and National Center for Assisted Living (AHCA-/NCAL, ahcancal.org)) found 94% of nursing home providers had staff shortages and more than half had lost key members of their staff during the pandemic due to workers quitting. The job is tough, and few want to endanger their lives and the lives of their families for what they were being paid. In some cases, the pay of those who worked in COVID units was increased. While many workers took the offer, others decided it wasn't worth the peril. "What you're telling nursing home assistants, nursing home staff, is that they need to work for probably the same amount of pay – or maybe a small raise, who knows – and they need to put their lives and their family's lives at risk by going into a nursing home where COVID-19 could creep in at any time," said an assistant professor of health policy and management cited in the CNN report. Nursing home staff across the country are demanding change and better pay and providers are calling on the government for more funding to tackle the staffing crisis.

Facilities that receive Medicaid and Medicare payments are required to provide 24-hour licensed nursing services, have a registered nurse for at least eight consecutive hours every day, and have a registered nurse designated to serve as director of nursing on a full-time basis. Yet there are no federal requirements for daily nursing hours per resident. In March 2021, the Health Affairs journal (healthaffairs.org) surmised that nationally, registered nurses in nursing homes had an average turnover rate of more than 140% in 2017 and 2018. Certified nursing aides had a turnover rate of more than 129%. Some facilities, the journal offered, had annual total nursing staff turnover rates of more than 300%.

The CNN report continues that while some Americans do pay for nursing homes on their own, most of the facilities' income comes from Medicaid and Medicare. Medicaid reimbursements, determined by each state, pay for long-stay residents, who make up the majority of the nursing home population, while Medicare reimburses facilities – at generally higher rates – for short-stay patients who are usually there for rehabilitation services. Difficult aspects of COVID in a nursing facility are not only isolation and the aforementioned concerns. What makes shortages of help worse is when sections of a facility are cordoned off, placing positive-testing residents in specific sections or isolating residents who have been in contact with positive staff members. To avoid cross-contamination, non-positive staff members are limited and confined to the COVID halls, unable to assist elsewhere in the building,

The AHCA/NCAL has been pushing for more funding for nursing homes, says the CNN report, especially for better Medicaid reimbursements from Congress and state governments. In March, 2021, President Joe Biden called on Congress to allocate $400 billion to expand access to affordable home- and community-based care.

Facility residents and staff have suffered and paid a high price to survive, keep themselves safe, and keep their families safe. The pandemic has put the spotlight on the need to improve services and increase staff in long-term facilities. The devastation has been egregious throughout the U.S. The Nursing Home Reform Modernization Act of 2020 would increase educational resources for those facilities that under-perform and establish an independent advisory council to inform the U.S. Department of Health and Human Services on how to further quality improvements.

What can you do? Advocate. Write or call your Members of Congress to urge passage of the Nursing Home Reform Modernization Act. Determining which nursing home is right for you or a loved one depends on resources to ensure that vulnerable seniors and veterans receive the quality of care they deserve. In a press release (December 18, 2020) from the office of Congresswoman Anna G. Eshoo in California's 18th Congressional District, Representative Eshoo has fought for better standards of care and infection control in long-term facilities. She introduced the Nursing Home COVID-19 Protection and Prevention Act 2020, designed to permit states to invest in "strike teams" of health care providers to assist when a COVID-19 outbreak happens. The Act would also provide for funding for staffing, testing, and personal protective equipment. The goal of this Coronavirus relief package is to stop COVID-19 infections and deaths among nursing home residents – and workers. The Act will demand accountability among nursing homes with the worst performances.

Know what is occurring with Congressional legislation that will benefit you and your loved ones now and in the future. Representative Eshoo, who also chairs the House Health Subcommittee said, "Over 200,000 long-term care residents and staff have died due to COVID-19. This staggering national tragedy requires immediate federal action to improve care and save lives in our nation's nursing homes." Passage of these bills and more like them will give seniors the power to choose a nursing home that is suitable and effective, and will help them live their golden days in peace, comfort, and without worry.

Again, advocate.

"The next time you see one of those beautiful buildings designed for the elderly or immobile, remember there are real people inside who need your support -- whether family, friends, or neighbors. Visit them, pray for them, advocate for them, and don't abandon them. They need your love, visits, and presence in their lives."
– Patricia Gunn, Esquire, Ohio University professor emerita and former caregiver for her mother

Chapter 28 – What I've Learned: Advocacy

When I began using a wheelchair on a more permanent basis in 2002, the reality of inaccessibility was prevalent at every turn – transportation, lodging, restaurants, stores, parking, classrooms, attitudes – everywhere. A colleague, who happens to be blind, and I advocated for change in myriad areas at our town and beyond, individually and through committees. I wrote letters to establishments and various venues (I have a file of nearly 50 letters) letting them know what worked and what didn't for a person with a disability, especially from where I sat. Advocacy works as gradual changes went into effect.

Whenever I teach a course, I ask at the beginning of each class "What are you thinking?" The responses I often hear are remarkable from, "I really want to get an 'A' in this course" and "I'm wondering if my assignments are complete" to "I need to call my mother" and "I forgot to put money in the meter." I excused the student to take care of his parking before he received a ticket. At the end of each class, I ask "What was your learning today?" Students need to pay attention because they never know whose name I will call to give a response for at least three things they learned in class that day. In all I try to accomplish, thinking through the process is important and then learning and taking away something from the experience is crucial.

What have I learned as an insider? I've learned advocacy by the person in a facility or hospital, if able, or by a family member, friend, caregiver, or health care provider is critical. My daughter is such an advocate for me and leaves no stone unturned. Again, the aides and the nurses would often ask, "Is your daughter coming in today?" I really didn't know because she just pops in at any time, day or night, so that she could see what was going on for herself. She had to, because I was so sick when I arrived I barely knew which way was up. She knows the way I like things and would let the staff, even the administrators, know what was working for me and what was not. You have to speak up.

The definition of advocacy is the act of speaking on behalf of or in support of another person, place, or thing. An example of an advocacy is a non-profit organization that works to help women of domestic abuse who feel too afraid to speak for themselves.

The qualities of a good healthcare advocate:

- Being assertive and comfortable talking with doctors and healthcare providers and getting them to answer questions in plain English (not medical terminology);
- Having the time to be at the facility which might be difficult for someone with a demanding job or family responsibilities;
- Being organized to help handle the paperwork and willing to take notes and gather information from the health care team about diagnosis and treatment; and
- Being someone who is comfortable with health details and with whom that information should be shared.

The main role of an advocate is to help lower the risk of medical errors and ensure the most appropriate care is received from qualified, experienced specialists and to make sure wishes are respected. An advocate should ask about follow-up care and recovery. When a patient is ready to be discharged from the facility or hospital, an advocate should ask the physician about the first follow-up visit and by whom, if any medications should be continued or discontinued, how to care for any incisions or wounds, if any special equipment is needed at home during recovery, if there are limitations on what can be done, and what symptoms could indicate a complication or side effect that requires more medical attention.

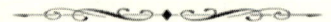

Chapter 29 – Observations Over My Six Nursing Home Journeys and My Recommendations

My observations represent those from the nursing homes (good, bad, and ugly) I've visited or in which I have been a resident, not just one specific facility.

Facility recommendations:

- Cleanliness is paramount, with no foul smells throughout the facility, especially at the entrance.
- Have tiled or wooden floors.
- Have individual rooms with private bathrooms and showers, even if it means renovating the facility. Privacy is essential.
- Provide good meals. We eat first with our eyes. Make it presentable and, above all, edible.
- Facilities need better security and cameras at doors, even outside.
- Utilize voicemail to allow messages to be left.

- Place white boards in rooms showing who is on the shifts.
- Include a therapy pool when constructing new facilities.

Administration and staff recommendations:
- Administrators should be accessible to staff and residents. Walk the halls. Be visible. Help when needed.
- Adequately and skillfully staff the facility. Those who hire should have keen human resources skills or human resources experience.
- Add more common use equipment, such as Hoyer lifts, sit-to-stands, physical/occupational therapy equipment, and vitals machines.
- Take the recommendations of therapists when equipment is needed to enhance residents' progress.
- Provide a thorough orientation to all employees. Most times, aides don't have a clue as to whom they should report. When I meet a new aide, I suggest things that will make them successful and that will help properly take care of the residents: Be cheerful; care for the people; anticipate needs; listen; be polite; answer call lights promptly; and don't disappear. Love residents (no matter how cantankerous they are) as you would your favorite grandparent.
- Some staff cheat the system by taking more than the allotted breaks and long lunches, while others are not able to take breaks at all.
- The "charge" nurse in charge should have management/leadership skills and have the authority to make decisions.
- Don't just hire a warm body. I have had plenty of them. Health care workers should be thoroughly vetted, trained, and oriented, and not let loose by themselves on a floor until they are ready. There should be regular oversight.
- Respect and appreciate all levels of staff and value their skills.

- Staff need "down time" – some are overworked and underpaid (aides).
- Have staff peep into rooms at the beginning of each shift to say hello. We often never know who is on the hall.
- When an employee is a bad one or walks off the job, let them go. Don't provide a good recommendation and don't rehire. Hire someone better.
- Don't play favorites to family members or friends. Other staff take notice of the difference which affects morale.
- Answer all call lights promptly, even if it's not your hall or the aide is not in your "clique."
- Nurses must help answer call lights when possible and must not be crude, "annoyed," or have attitudes. My peeve is when nurses will look for an aide to respond to a call light and not answer it themselves if the aide is busy. I've seen nurses chatting and simply ignoring lights. I was told by an administrator that no one in the facility – no one – should pass a light without responding for the resident might be in distress. They might not be able to help but can let someone know the person's status.
- Teamwork must be woven into the fabric of a nursing home. Staff should not have the luxury to decide other staff members they will or will not assist or what residents they will or will not assist. You're in the wrong business without teamwork.
- When hiring STNAs and nurses who are still in school or taking courses to advance themselves, remember that and schedule with compassion. Be flexible and good people will work even harder for the facility and its residents. If not, they are gone.
- Staff should leave attitudes and problems at home. We residents already have enough of our own.
- So, what if you're having a bad day or had trouble at home. Don't be abrasive to other employees and talk down to them. Treat others as you want to be treated.

- Don't talk about all you have to do and then rush when helping. It makes residents think they are less than important than the next one.
- Don't talk about other staff or residents, even if you think no one is listening. We hear you. If you talk about them, you will talk about us.
- If you have been an aide or a nurse before coming to a new facility, fine. Don't tell residents about your prior history and proceed as if you know it all. Every facility, room, resident, and procedure is different. Listen and learn before making assumptions.
- Emphasize the importance of staff friendliness to residents, family members, visitors, and to each other. Favor patients over paperwork. (Again, I was neglected too long on a few occasions by a nurse who said her "paperwork was important." When she finally came to me, I asked her what was the priority there, paperwork or patient work? Needless to say, I left that facility as soon as possible.) At another facility, I observed a nurse pointing her finger in the face of a resident, who often presented herself as needy and pesky. The nurse telling the resident she didn't have time to deal with her. It's often not what you say, but how you say it. Model customer service and kindness.
- Keep vigilant about wound prevention and wound care. Wounds are easy to get and difficult to heal. I got three terrible wounds at one facility. My wounds got so bad over time that one was infected almost to the bone. Today, two wounds are healed and the other has gone from the size of a baseball to the size of a dime. The current facility has done a phenomenal job getting me healed and scheduling me for an excellent wound care clinic in Lancaster, Ohio. Everyone needs to know the value and necessity of protein in the healing process. I didn't understand that at first.
- Most aides are often not respected by some nurses. Listen to aides and don't so easily dismiss what they are saying. Aides have their fingers on the pulse and know residents better than anyone.

- Residents suffer when staff is short or is not trustworthy. Consider a shower aide and/or a float aide for the busiest shifts.
- Stress the importance of family support – over and over and over. The loss of socialization and not seeing family during COVID caused many residents to quickly go downhill.
- Survival in a nursing facility depends on attitude, support, social activities, therapy, medical care, and diet. Plus, helping residents and staff maintain positive attitudes; "can do" attitudes go a long way toward mental and physical stability.
- Reward those at a facility who are dedicated, loyal, make extra efforts, and are good at what they do. Fire the ones who aren't, especially if they are only working for a paycheck. Don't retain those who act as if they would rather be somewhere else or are talking/texting on their phones or getting cozy in a resident's room without permission, e.g., sitting/sleeping on the couch, sitting in the resident's wheelchair or on the bed.
- Staff who work with residents must be caring, kind, and patient. Never yell at residents – or each other. Praise publicly; criticize privately.
- Don't let the rumor mill become your downfall or add to it. Believe none of what you hear and only half of what you see.
- Use People First language. All too often I hear from aides or nurses, "I've got 'a feed' or I've got a 'wheelchair'." Instead say, "I've got a 'person' to feed," or "I have to get 'someone' in a wheelchair." Not using people-first language reduces residents to objects.
- Preach and model kindness.

Policy recommendations:
- If policies and procedures are followed daily, there is no need to panic when Corporate or State come for an

inspection or a visit. Everyone shows up, helps, and responds to call lights then.

- Permit unlimited family and friends' access with appropriate security and health precautions.
- A facility needs to help people, not count pennies and scrimp on supplies, food, and other essentials.
- Needed is an overhaul of the health care system for equity in pay, care, insurance, cost of care in facilities and hospitals, cost of medications, transportation consideration, the eternal need for "productivity," and the cost of care and treatment.

I was FaceTiming with my daughter the day before Thanksgiving 2020 when we heard a commotion in the room next to me and someone yelling at a resident. Because the resident was extremely needy and could be trying, the nurse lost her patience and raised her voice at him. She then slammed his door. My daughter said, "Is that someone speaking to you like that?" I said, "No, it's (nurse's name) speaking to the resident next door," My daughter, ever the advocate, said, "Let me speak with the nurse." I told her I would handle it, being the advocate I've become. When the nurse came back down the hall, I called her in the room and said, as I have said to her before, "Be kind, be kind, be kind" and reminded her that these were the three principles of Mister Rogers of Mister Rogers' Neighborhood on PBS. I can't stress these principles enough in all areas of your life. He listed them as, "number one, be kind; number two, be kind; and, by now, you know what the third is? Be kind." I admonished her that, except for the grace of God, that resident – who had a brain injury –

might be her in 20 or 30 years. Except for the grace of God, there we go.

That resident died the next day due to health complications. (Several months later, the nurse – who was always full of drama – was dismissed for not doing her job properly, not because of the death, but for other reasons.)

"Kindness is the language which the deaf can hear and the blind can see." – Mark Twain

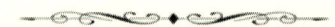

Chapter 30 – Touching Lives

I'm here to witness and, while here, I'll heal.

I had an aide who, believe it or not, seemed to be avoiding me. She would be otherwise occupied when it was time to handle my care and would send someone else. One day, I said, "You aren't present for me." She quietly said, "Did someone say something to you?" I said, "No." She thought someone had mentioned her past with Black people. Again, I said, "No." I added, "Why would you think that and have I treated you any differently?" She came to my side and shared her story with apologetic tears. Her ancestors, she explained, had been involved in lynching a Black man. For some reason, she thought I knew that. She apologized over and over, asking for forgiveness and cried. I told her she was not responsible for their actions and what she needed to do going forward was to love everyone regardless of color or creed and to be the difference in her family and in her community. I was able to explain history from 1619 and what has occurred with my people over the years, and today – how the enslaved built the U.S. economy by the sweat of their brow while being lynched, beaten, raped, and separated from families. The summer that Mr. George Floyd was murdered unfortunately afforded me the opportunity to explain why we march and what it's like in America to walk, drive, or even live while Black. Telling the story over and over to those who asked was exhausting, but so very necessary.

Another aide was having difficulty passing the test to become a licensed practical nurse. After many "encouragement" sessions, I helped her with a plan of action and with developing a study schedule. Her confidence was low, and my daughter and I worked with her on boosting that level and helping her realize she could do this. After much prayer and study, she took the test again and she gave us the news. She passed and, just as she was a great and compassionate aide, she is a great nurse. She does not let the degree stop her from helping when needed in a room, even if "it is not a nurse's job" as a few nurses say. She does not call someone else to help when she is right there to assist. I know she will make an excellent registered nurse one day.

A very demure young man, with little confidence, was introduced to me. He was a new aide. I liked him from the start as he was polite and seemed to want to do a great job for those in his care. As I usually do, I asked questions about his life and goals. Over time, he confided in me that he was homeless and he, and his parents, had been living out of their vehicles. I began to pray for him, learned he had faith in God and was a genuinely good, solid person. He just had some bad breaks in life. He met the right person. Me. I encouraged him in confidence building and prompted him to work toward a degree one day. He started to save his money and now has an apartment for him and his family. He's also pursuing another career.

As I was making the edits to this book, sitting in the activities room, in walked a new hire in activities and said I was just the person she needed to see. She asked if I remembered her. I have to say, I didn't at first until I peeped at her badge. "You're the reason I'm here," she said. I looked at her puzzled. She continued, "I came to work in 2019 with housekeeping and I was doing my duties in a room when I come across you. We got to talking and you asked me if I knew where I was headed in life and about plans that I had for my future.

"As we talked, I realized that I wasn't in the place that I needed to be in, that I wasn't living to my full potential. I started to dig deeper inside my own thoughts and feelings and realized you were on to something – I wasn't living my life to the fullest and wasn't where or what I was meant to be.

"After a year of traveling around trying to find my place in this world and being very unsuccessful, I found myself re-applying to this facility. In August 2020, I was offered my position back with housekeeping and shortly after that realized I still wasn't where I was meant to be. So, I did some more searching and, within two days, I found my place in activities. It has opened me up so much to where I want to be. I am finally getting to care for people one-on- one. It's not just about cleaning a room or straightening or even dusting; it's about the care of the resident and when I come into a room now, I don't bring a quart of cleaning supplies. I bring smiles. I bring conversation. I bring help and love what I do for once in my life.

"The day you prayed for me changed my life. As of October 1, 2020, I will officially begin my dream job as an STNA. I cannot thank anyone for this except you. I will go into this journey wholeheartedly and I will be grateful every single day for your helping me finally find the path I was meant to be on. I would not be here if it was not for you. I really want things in the world so that I can genuinely say my children are proud of me again. In 33 years, no one encouraged me and I am forever indebted to you. Last, but not least, when I wake up in the morning I wake up with purpose. I put my feet on the floor with a smile and I'm ready to go to work and do my job the way God wanted me to do. If it wasn't for you seriously having that one-on-one conversation with a complete stranger, I would probably still be lost – I would be wandering out there somewhere."

She explained to me that she was angry with God because she felt like He took her mother, her best friend, and her aunt. She said until she met me, she never saw any light in her life, but I gave her purpose. She said I gave her a reason to keep going because she went to drinking for three years and, finally, when my words kept ringing in her ears and then she saw me in a video promoting the facility, she said her whole family sat there and cheered because she talked about me and the influence I had been in her life. "I'm on the right road now," she said as she smiled. "I'm taking this journey one step at a time."

She's got a wonderful relationship with her children and her husband is her rock. Her son is a great football player, her daughter plays volleyball, and she just sees her life with a new direction. She said no one had ever spoken life or light into her life and it makes her life worth living. She added, "It is rare to find people who don't always think about themselves."

This is when I had to tell her about my life with my Mama Thelma, how she raised me, how she always gave, and thought about others before herself. When there was a death in the community or in the church, she was there to provide a meal or some kind of financial support. She was a listening ear. She was everybody's Mama. More importantly, she was my great aunt and raised me as her own when my mother and father could not care for me.

As I was close to publishing, I received a phone call from a young lady I mentored at a facility. A month or so earlier, she told me she was planning to interview for a job and wasn't certain about how she should go about it. I asked her about the position and, right on the spot, I conducted a mock interview with her and gave her tips on the process. When the opportunity arose to provide a reference, I did that. I made myself available to her to calm any fears and to give encouragement. Back to the call – she was offered the position! I've never heard anyone so appreciative and grateful. All I ever ask in return is that the recipient of the blessing give God the glory and pay it forward.

These stories are only five among many, but they all deal with one thing: Purpose. Everything we do in life is not always pleasant yet, if we can see past ourselves and our fears, we can understand that there's purpose not just for ourselves, but also for someone else. I've been in such homes and centers for such a time as this – placed exactly where God wanted me. My professor friend always reminds me that in God, things always work out the way they are supposed to be.

I've learned through my health experiences that life is not what I expected. It's tough. I was experiencing some really rough marital issues in 1974. My pastor's wife in Morgantown would always tell me, "Honey, just hang in there because you're going to come out as pure gold and you're going be able to help somebody else." In my despair, I thought, "What in the world is she talking about?" I thought I couldn't ever help anybody going through this myself, but I learned if you hang in there long enough and trust God, you can make it. It's the same with my health and having to spend so much time in facilities away from my home.

No one but God knows the tears and how I've cried out to Him to increase my mobility, give me more independence, heal the wounds, and get me home. During good weather, one of my favorite things to do is go outside, feel the sun on my face, look at the puffy cloud formations, listen to the birds, and talk to God. Of course, I talk to Him in my room and elsewhere, but there's something about the outdoors that makes me feel closer to His presence.

After praying and praying and praying, I'm still here – in a facility – 2021. I think about this little cartoon character named Shorty McShort Short who tells people that, no matter what, to keep on keeping on. I have been to church services where the healing anointing was strong and I knew I would get up out of the wheelchair and walk. People have prayed and are still praying for me to walk on my own. I'm still here. Yes, purpose.

My professor friend recounted a situation when, during a church service, the minister announced his eyes were healed. My friend, who was blind from birth, said his grandmother pulled him up and took him out of the service. He remembers the number of times people proclaimed his healing, but God did not see it that way and his grandmother knew it. This gentleman happens to be a phenomenal person, husband, father, preacher, professor, author, musician, mentor, and advocate who stands on God's Word in that, "His grace is sufficient for you, for My power is made perfect in weakness. Therefore, I will boast the more gladly about my weaknesses, so that Christ's power may rest in me" (2 Corinthians 12:9). He preaches about the Apostle Paul's thorn in the flesh that God did not remove, but Paul had to live with it – certainly discomfort and all whether physical or spiritual. My friend says he doesn't know how he would be with sight, that some things, temporary or permanent, come to keep us humble and grounded. No matter if God does or does not heal, He is still able to do so!

A Nigerian student with a disability came to the university in a broken down wheelchair. She could not walk and had deformed hands. I asked her how she could persevere with the condition of her chair and the campus not so accommodating at the time. She said, "You know what? If you can't go on under it, you have to go over; if you can't go through, go around; if you can't go over it, go under it." She earned her master's degree and gave me a life lesson.

Her story still stays with me today after more than 20 years. It all boils down to purpose – the reason something is done or created or for which something exists. Mark Twain said the two most important days in your life are the day you are born and the day you find out why.

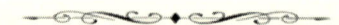

Chapter 31 – Reflections

As I reflect on my "insider's" experiences in and out of rehabilitation facilities over the years and going through physical, and other therapies, recovering, setbacks, hospital visits, and needing care to rehabilitate my body, I may have had my moments but always looked up to God from whence comes my help (Psalm 121:1). When I might have been having a moment, someone would come to me for prayer, uplifting, advice, encouragement in school to push themselves beyond what they think they can do, or just plain survival tips. Again, I refused to let someone come in my room who was staff saying they were just okay or having a bad day. I would simply say, "Look around you. You have a job, you are walking, talking, and lucid. You're not in this bed or in a room. You can come and go, Consider the alternative," ("and shut up!"). They would perk up with my subtle attitude adjustment. It gives me joy because

I know my life has purpose as I've given other people purpose through their (and my) pain in these hospitals and facilities over the years.

One Sunday, I filled in for Pastor Bolin at Romans Road Church and I talked about how those of us present had made it through COVID when so many others did not. I spoke about how we need each other to survive. A facility will test residents' memory by asking them to recall three words. I highlighted words that we should speak to each other, how we should pray for, love, and treat those around us kindly because we need each other to survive in this world. The next day, a gentleman who attended and who had difficulty filtering his words, came to my door and said he wanted to give his life to the Lord. Purpose.

I defied the odds in 1995 when the doctors didn't think I would live through an 11-hour operation to remove the spinal cord tumor. I not only walked again, but I thrived and survived. I have spoken life into others through God who gives me and everyone life.

This is a part of my journey but not the end because I have many things yet to accomplish and people to inspire. I will continue working hard in physical therapy because, speaking those things that are not as though they are, I will regain mobility and return to my earthly home. I will continue to enjoy life, my family, and living. I will continue to strive to be a blessing and to be one of God's change agents.

The care and dedication of anyone who works in any aspect of health care cannot be underestimated. These are people from housekeeping and laundry to aides, nurses, doctors, and administrators who, for the most part, give their all every day to ensure residents and patients are cared for appropriately.

To all who have helped me in any way: Thank you. To those who slacked, misrepresented me, or just didn't care – not only for me, but for others as well: I forgive you. Just be better and do better.

"I'll get you through and I'll get you to your home," God reminds me.

"Right now, though, you're walking and working in My purpose."

Resources

Affordable Care Act, 2010. Retrieved from
    www.healthcare.gov.

American Health Care Association and National Center
    for Assisted Living. Retrieved from www.ahcancal.org.

Athens News. (2019, March 25). Ohio Health. Canine Care:
    Therapy Dogs Program Launches at O'Bleness Hospital.
    Retrieved from www.athensnews.com.

CMS Nursing Home Data Compendium. (2010).
    American Nurses Association.
    Retrieved from www.nursingworld.org/practice-pol-
    icy/workforce/what-is-nursing/.

Center, N. H. A. (2016, March 30). Elder Abuse Statistics –
    Statistics on Elderly Abuse Over Time.
    Retrieved from www.nursinghomeabusecenter.com/el-
    der-abuse/statistics/.

Centers for Disease Control and Prevention.
    (2021, January 13). Nursing Homes and Long-Term
    Care. Retrieved from www.cdc.gov.

Centers for Disease Control and Prevention. (2021, March 3).
    Older Adult Falls. Retrieved from www.cdc.gov.

Centers for Medicare & Medicare Services.
    Retrieved from www.cms.gov.

Elder Abuse. Retrieved from
    www.who.int/news-room/fact-sheets/detail/elder-
    abuse.

Eshoo, Pascrell, Kelly, McKinley Lead Critical Legislation to Reform Nursing Home Care Amid Pandemic. (2020, December 18). Retrieved from www.eshoo.house.gov.

Genworth Cost of Care Survey. (2020, December 2). Retrieved from www.genworth.com.

Harrington, C., Corrillo, H., Garfield, R., & Squires, E. (2018, April 3). Nursing Facilities, Staffing, Residents, and Facility Deficiencies, 2009 through 2016. Retrieved from www.kff.org.

Health Affairs. (2021, March). Retrieved from www.healthaffairs.org.

History of Physical Therapy. (2020, October 6). Retrieved from www.jointventurespt.com.

House Finance Agencies. Retrieved from www.ncshs.org.

Nursing Home Reform Modernization Act, S.4866), 2020. Retrieved from www.aging.senate.gov.

Jaffe, I. (2017, August 28). Serious Nursing Home Abuse Often Not Reported to Police, Federal Investigators Find. Retrieved from www.npr.org/2017/08/28/546460187/serious-nursing-home-abuse-often-not-reported-to-police-federal-inves-tigators-fi.

Justice for Nursing Home Abuse. (2019, January 7). Statistics on Nursing Home Abuse – Get the Facts You Need. Retrieved from www.justiceforelderabuse.com.

King James Bible. (1962). Thompson Chain Reference, Zondervan.

King James Bible. (2020). King James Bible Online: www.kingjamesbibleonline.org.

Lewis, C. (2020. May 21). COVID-19: An Insider's Look at Skilled Care. Retrieved from www.athensmessenger.com.

Maxouris, C. (2021, July 6). Covid-19 Exposed the Devastating Consequences of Staff Shortages in Nursing Homes. But the Problem Isn't New. Retrieved from www.cnn.com/2021/06/27/us/nursinghomes-staff-shortages/index.html.

MetLife Market Survey of Long-Term Care Costs. (2012). Retrieved from www.theceal.com.

Moninger, M. (2019, September 9). A Brief History of Occupational Therapy. Retrieved from www.myotspot.com.

National Association of Social Workers. (2003). NASW Standards for Social Work Services in Long-Term Care Facilities. Retrieved from www.socialworkers.org.

National Center for Victims of Crime. Retrieved from www.victimsofcrime.org.

Nursing Home Abuse Center. Retrieved from www.nursinghomeabusecenter.com.

Nursing Home Care. Centers for Disease Control and Prevention. Retrieved from www.cdc.gov.

Nursing Home Reform Act, 1987. Retrieved from www.aarp.org.

Older Americans Act, 1965. Retrieved from www.acl.gov.

Rau, J., & Leeds, A. (2018, July 13). Like a Ghost Town: Erratic Nursing Home Staffing Revealed Through New Records. Keyser Health News. Retrieved from www.khn.org.

The Canadian Press. (2019, February 6). Police Called to Bingo Game Brawl at Long-Term Care Home. Retrieved from www.beta.ctvnews.ca.

The Nursing Home COVID-19 Protection and Prevention Act. (2020). Retrieved from www.eshoo.house.gov.

U.S. Bureau of Labor Statistics. Retrieved from www.bls.gov.

Winner-Swete, T. (2014, April 21). Bingo: A Cultural and Generational Experience. Retrieved from www.museumofplay.org.

World Health Organization, (2021, June 15). Elder Abuse. Retrieved from www.who.int/news-room/fact-sheets/detail/elder-abuse.

About the Author

Dr. Carolyn Bailey Lewis retired from public media in 2011 following a distinguished 38-year career. Her most recent position was as director and general manager of WOUB Public Media at Ohio University in Athens where she served for 13 years as the first woman and first Black person to lead this entity and the first woman to be Emerita. She was also general manager at WNPB-TV in Morgantown, West Virginia, and was the first Black woman to head a public television station in the continental United States (1994). She is the recipient of numerous awards and honors, including industry and university awards for professional achievement. Dr. Lewis has served as a consultant to public television stations, is a sought-after speaker and presenter, and was elected or appointed to numerous national and state public media committees and boards, including the Association of Public Television Stations' Board of Trustees in D.C. and the Sesame Workshop in New York City. She established a scholarship for students at WOUB. Dr. Lewis taught in the Perley I. Reed School of Journalism (now Reed College of Media) at West Virginia University (WVU), the Scripps College of Communication at Ohio University, and is an adjunct professor for Hocking College. She serves on several local and state committees, is a member of Alpha Kappa Alpha Sorority, Incorporated, and is an ordained minister. She earned bachelor's and master's degrees in journalism from WVU in Morgantown, the first Black woman to graduate with an undergraduate degree in journalism (1971), and she earned a Ph.D. in Communication Studies from the Scripps College of Communication at Ohio University. Her dissertation, "Identity: Lost, Found, and (Re)constructed – An Autoethnography of Tragedy, Travail, and Triumph," can be found at
https://search.proquest.com/open-
view/ab58c6459a39df30e62c20c029bc038d/1pqorig
site=gscholar&cbl=18750&diss=y.

Dr. Lewis is an advocate for accessibility and inclusion, serving as a consultant on those issues. She and her daughter Caryn M. Bailey, MPA, Major Giving Officer and an OHIO doctoral student, are co-founders of the Dr. Carolyn Foster Bailey Lewis Family Foundation, a charitable organization which promotes health, wellness, and education for those with acute and chronic illnesses, and disabilities (www.drcarolynfosterbaileylewisff.org). A portion of the proceeds of this book will assist the work of the Foundation. They also co-founded LifeDay Greeting Cards, Inc., unique greeting cards celebrating life and survival of life-altering events (www.lifedaygreetingcards.com).

Contact Information
carolyn@drcarolynfosterbaileylewisff.org

Made in United States
North Haven, CT
02 December 2021

11871758R00140